"*Healing the Sick Care System carries a deeply human voice. Gil Bashe draws on the grit of someone who has spent a lifetime inside the system to show where we fall short and where hope still lives. His stories don't lecture; they illuminate. They reveal how care actually feels when you're the one in the room and why the system so often forgets that simple truth. This book makes a compelling case for putting people back at the center of medicine, delivered with honesty and empathy that stays with you.*"

– John Nosta

Author, Speaker, Global Innovation Theorist,
and Psychology Today Columnist

"*In a world where we assume technology is the answer to fixing healthcare, Gil Bashe brings forth a different paradigm—putting the patient at the center and leading with empathy. Through Gil's experiences as a medical professional, policy leader, clergy, patient, and patient advocate, he shares heartfelt and poignant stories that underscore the need to move forward using technology and a human-centered, empathetic approach to care. This is a powerful must-read for anyone eager to effect change in our health system.*"

– Sally Ann Frank

Global Lead, Health & Life Sciences,
Microsoft for Startups, Microsoft

"*This book is for everyone who believes we can do better. It exposes the cracks in our sick-care system, but more importantly, it shows how each of us—patients, providers, payers, policymakers, and innovators—can become part of the solution. If you care about the future of health(care), you'll find both urgency and hope in these pages.*"

– Daniel Kraft, MD

Founder, NextMed Health
and Digital.Health

"*Gil Bashe is the insider willing to name where the system fails patients and exactly who must take responsibility.* Healing the Sick Care System *challenges leaders to stop hiding behind process and own the human consequences of the decisions they approve.*"

– Matthew Zachary

Founder, Stupid Cancer;
Host, Out of Patients Podcast

"*Gil Bashe knows the U.S. medical system both professionally and as the father of a child with a rare disease. His book is a moving cri de coeur about the dysfunction of this system, which features the most advanced medical treatment and drug innovation in the world, yet makes it difficult or impossible for many of its citizens to gain access to them.*"

– Ron Cohen, MD

Biopharma Founder, Chief Executive, and
Board Director, Egret Therapeutics

"*Gil Bashe cuts through the noise of our fractured system to remind us that patients deserve care rooted in evidence and empathy. His insights expose how structural barriers undermine progress in chronic conditions like obesity, where misinformation and delayed access can cost lives. This book is a timely call to redesign care so that every person receives the thoughtful, science-based support they need to achieve lasting health."*

– Katherine H. Saunders, MD

Co-Founder, Flytehealth; Clinical Assistant Professor of Medicine, Weill Cornell Medicine

"Healing the Sick Care System *is a timely reminder that innovation means little unless it reaches people and improves their lives. Gil Bashe challenges us to pair scientific progress with empathy, accountability, and a renewed commitment to those we serve. This book resonates with the Galien Foundation's mission: advancing breakthroughs that honor humanity as much as they honor science."*

– Bruno Cohen

Chairman,
Galien Foundation

"*When bureaucracy eclipses compassion, lives hang in the balance. Packed with insight, urgency, and vision,* Healing the Sick Care System *is for anyone who believes that life—and the care we give one another—matters most. It is a call to action, a guide, and a blueprint for transforming a fragmented healthcare system into one that honors the people it exists to serve."*

– Michael L. Weamer

President and CEO,
The Marfan Foundation

" Healing the Sick Care System: Why People Matter *is the wake-up call every patient and care partner has been waiting for. This book returns humanity to the center of medicine, reminding us that behind every test result, every diagnosis, every policy, every prior authorization, there is a person who needs and deserves to be seen, heard, and treated with dignity. Read it and join the movement to build a care system that answers to its most important customer: you."*

– Grace Cordovano, PhD

Founder, Enlightening Results;
Co-Founder, Unblock Health

" *Gil Bashe takes a clear-eyed look at what is working, and what is failing, in the U.S. health system. Drawing on experiences that span from his early days carrying punch cards as a graduate student to decades as a global health leader, he shows why health must be built around people, not just process. Having taught more than 10,000 graduate and executive education students in the U.S. and India over three decades, Bashe offers a timely and valuable read for both new and experienced health leaders."*

– Stan Kachnowski, PhD, MPA

Co-Founder and Chairman, HITLAB
(Health Innovation Technology Lab)

" *In a time when medicine grows more complex by the day, this book powerfully reaffirms the physician's role as a trusted partner in every person's health journey. Gil Bashe reminds us that healing begins with listening, collaboration, and compassion. His insights champion a system where health professionals and patients work side by side to achieve better outcomes and a better care experience."*

– John Whyte, MD, MPH

Author; CEO and Executive Vice President,
American Medical Association

"With early grounding on the battlefield dealing with life-and-death situations as a medic, Gil Bashe grew up to champion the Global Health and Purpose Practices at FINN Partners. His pivot from 'battlefield to boardroom' eventually led him to a higher calling—a call to action—to collaborate across our special interests, united for patients: consumers, caregivers, and citizens. In Healing the Sick Care System: Why People Matter, *Gil shares insightful, hard-hitting anecdotes and hard data that, woven together, inspire us to imagine, design, and rebuild a health ecosystem for all."*

– Jane Sarasohn-Kahn, MA, MHSA

Health Economist, Advisor,
Trend Weaver

"I met Gil Bashe more than three decades ago, and even then, he was already a leading communicator in the fields of health and wellness. What makes Gil unique is that he approaches every challenge with the patient at the forefront of his thinking. This book reflects that commitment. It is grounded in a clear understanding of the complexities of the American health system and a genuine empathy for the obstacles consumers and health professionals face as they try to navigate it. He champions a patient-centric approach that is essential to improving health outcomes."

– Paul Holmes

Founder, CEO, and Editor-in-Chief,
PRovoke Media

HEALING THE SICK CARE SYSTEM
Why People Matter

Copyright © 2026, **Gil Bashe**

Published by:
ThoughtLeaderPress.com

All rights reserved.

No part of this publication may be reproduced, stored in a retrieval system, stored in a database and / or published in any form or by any means, electronic, mechanical, photocopying, recording or otherwise, without the prior written permission of the author.

For the purpose of consistency, the publisher has often chosen to spell healthcare as one word.

First Edition

Ebook ISBN: 978-1-61343-182-5

Paperback ISBN: 978-1-61343-181-8

Hardcover ISBN: 978-1-61343-180-1

Healing the Sick Care System

Why People Matter

GIL BASHE

TABLE OF CONTENTS

FOREWORD

IN Health Care Nation, I wrote that we are living through the most consequential transformation in the history of modern medicine—a shift driven not by technology alone, but by a society finally waking up to the reality that our health system has become more "sick-care" than healthcare. We spend more, achieve less, and tolerate outcomes that would be unacceptable in every other industrialized nation. And because the system is strained, misaligned, and inequitable, the people inside it—clinicians, caregivers, patients—carry the burden.

That is why this book matters.

Gil Bashe has long been one of the clearest, most principled voices calling out the broken incentives and moral hazards that shape American healthcare. He has also been a persistent advocate for something our system desperately needs: a renewed social contract—one that treats health not as a commodity, but as a shared human responsibility.

What Gil has done here is more than diagnose what's wrong. He has written a book about possibility.

He reminds us that healthcare isn't failing because we lack clinical talent, scientific brilliance, or technological innovation. Healthcare is failing because the system around all that brilliance has calcified. Complexity has replaced clarity. Competition has replaced collaboration. Incentives reward activity, not outcomes. Stakeholders talk past one another. And the people we claim to serve increasingly feel unseen, unheard, and left to fend for themselves.

Gil brings a rare combination of moral conviction and industry fluency to these issues. He writes with the compassion of someone who has seen too many patients harmed by systemic inertia; with the clarity of someone who has worked across every part of the healthcare ecosystem; and with the urgency of someone who knows that incremental reform is no longer enough.

The Moment We Are In

We are now at an inflection point. Clinical workforce burnout is at record levels. Trust in health institutions is frayed. Chronic disease continues to rise. Communities with the least resources have the worst outcomes. And the economic strain of healthcare is no longer an isolated policy problem—it is a national security threat, a workforce threat, and a generational threat.

At the same time, we stand on the edge of unprecedented opportunity. Advances in artificial intelligence, predictive analytics, personalized medicine, and digital care delivery hold the potential to fundamentally rebalance how care is delivered. In the right hands and applied the right way, these tools can increase the human capacity to care for patients. They can reduce cognitive burden, eliminate waste, and restore clinicians to the work of healing.

But technology alone will not save us. Gil reminds us that tools don't transform systems—people and leadership do.

A System That Works for People, Not the Other Way Around

Throughout this book, Gil calls for something that should be obvious, but still isn't: healthcare must be designed around people—patients and professionals—not around payment models, regulatory structures, or institutional self-protection.

He challenges us to confront the uncomfortable truth that our system was never truly designed; it was assembled over decades, patchwork on top of patchwork. And now, as pressures mount, we see the consequences everywhere: from families who can't access basic care to nurses who can't take a lunch break to patients navigating a labyrinth of prior authorizations, portals, apps, and payer rules.

Gil's work is powerful because it rejects the false choice between moral purpose and operational excellence. He understands that doing the right thing and doing the smart thing are often the same. A system built around prevention costs less. A system built around trust works better. A system built around collaboration scales faster. A system built around health—rather than sick care—produces stronger, more resilient communities.

This is where his thinking aligns with the themes I explored in Health Care Nation: the recognition that change is not only possible, but necessary—and that the path forward requires courage, leadership, and a willingness to think boldly about what healthcare should be.

A Call to Action

What I admire most about Gil's writing is that he treats readers as partners in change. He doesn't offer passive commentary. He issues a call to action.

He asks leaders to rise above their institutional interests. He asks policymakers to prioritize health over politics. He asks clinicians to reclaim their voice and agency. He asks innovators to pursue progress with responsibility and humility. He asks all of us—citizens, consumers, communities—to demand better and imagine more.

Healthcare transformation is not theoretical. It is personal. Every one of us will eventually confront the system Gil describes—whether as a patient, a parent, a caregiver, or a loved one. And each of us has a role in shaping what comes next.

Why This Book Matters Now

This book arrives at precisely the right moment. It challenges the status quo with moral clarity. It reframes healthcare not as an industry, but as a shared human enterprise. It gives leaders a roadmap and citizens a voice. And it insists that the future is not something we wait for—it is something we build.

Gil Bashe has written a book full of truth, challenge, and hope. It forces us to reckon with what healthcare has become—and to imagine what it could be.

If you care about the future of American healthcare, read this book. And more importantly, act on it.

— **Tom Lawry**

Author, *Health Care Nation: The Future Is Calling and It's Better Than You Think*

ACKNOWLEDGMENTS

THIS book is the product of many voices, experiences, and moments of grace along the way. These ideas were not created in isolation but grew from countless interactions, lessons, and acts of support and kindness.

Family. First and always, I thank my family. My wife and daughter, both mental health professionals and writers, have been with me at every moment. They read through these pages, bringing their life experiences to bear, and encouraged me to advocate for everyone who enters the health system. They are my biggest fans and the foundation upon which I stand. To my grandmother, Ruth Bashe, whose endurance, having gone through fire and water, inspired me to find resilience when things looked dim. Her faith in me became the bedrock of my early confidence.

My appreciation to my late parents, Lila and Jerry Bashe, who brought me into the world, and whose end-of-life journeys strengthened my understanding of how we must confront the biology of disease and the obstacles of bureaucracy. I also honor the memory of my late father-in-law, Dr. Burt Giges, whose wide understanding of medicine and life's wisdom were precious jewels. I often think, "What would Burt do?" and still draw strength from that question, as well as from our enduring connection.

Foundations in Service. My foundational learning about medicine and addressing people's urgent health needs came from my military experience. I entered as a young, untested airborne medic and emerged as a seasoned veteran. My gratitude goes to all those I served with, and especially to my battalion commander and medical officer, for investing in me, trusting me, and shaping the discipline and compassion I have carried forward into every chapter of my career.

Mentors, Colleagues, and Leaders. I owe much to those who gave me guidance and opportunity. To Nick Adkins, Junaid Bajwa, MD, Bruno Cohen, Ron Cohen, MD, Edward Cox, Yael Elish, Sally Ann Frank, David Farber, Stef Guenther Kuhner, Stacy Hurt, Dr. Amir Kalali, Craig Lipset, Gregg Masters, Jane Sarasohn-Kahn, Mike Rea, Levi Shapiro, Matt Veatch, John Whyte, MD, Hal Wolf, and industry friends for contributing their encouragement and comments in support of this work. To Peter Finn, who encouraged me to think deeply about purpose and leadership. To the champions of patient advocacy organizations, especially Michael Weamer, who paved the way for me to take senior leadership roles within the American Heart Association and the Marfan Foundation. To my sounding board and guide, John Nosta, who continually challenges me to expand my perspective. To Tom Lawry, who is a thought partner and ally in advancing a patient-centered health system, and the generous author of the Foreword that affirms our shared mission. To colleagues at FINN Partners and throughout the agency's Health and Purpose Practices, whose friendship and counsel propel me to reach higher. To the many health-sector leaders mentioned throughout this book, my thanks for your constant collaboration and commitment to making the world healthier.

Friends and Communities. I am grateful to John Bianchi, Aleck McCathie and Christina Raish, who offered honest critique, editorial support, and encouragement when I needed it most. I also draw strength from the communities I have been privileged to be part of, including the Breslov Research Institute, CNS Summit, DTRA.org, the Galien Foundation, Healthcare NOW Radio, HIMSS, HITLAB, HLTH, Kibbutz Harel, Medika Life, Swaay, and ViVE. Your collective wisdom and camaraderie have shaped my journey.

Patients, Providers, and Advocates. My deepest gratitude to the patients, physicians, advocates, and organizations that have invited me to serve on their advisory boards, whose stories are woven into this book. You remind me that medicine is not only about

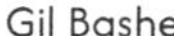

science, but also about meaning, trust, and humanity. Medicine is ultimately for the people.

Even the Obstacles. I also want to acknowledge those whose resistance or challenges compelled me to rethink, listen differently, and grow. Obstacles became lessons, and lessons became higher ground. For that, I am grateful.

With Gratitude to So Many. I cannot possibly name everyone who has shaped this journey; please know that even if not written here, your imprint is woven into these pages and into my heart.

To the Reader. Finally, to you, the reader. You chose to open this book because you care about the future of our health system. I hope that the ideas here affirm your role in helping us transform sick care into healthcare. If we rally to heal the system, we can do so much more for every person seeking healing.

INTRODUCTION

"HOUSTON, we have a problem."

Launched on April 11, 1970, Apollo 13 was to have been NASA's third lunar landing. Two days into the mission, an oxygen tank exploded, forcing the crew to abandon their plans to walk on the moon and focus on new goals: survival and return to Earth. The explosion crippled their capsule, but critically, it did not silence the radio connection. Because of the open link with Mission Control, the crew was able to assess and solve their problems and develop a plan to bring their command module safely home.

Were it not for that communication system, astronauts Jim Lovell, Jack Swigert, and Fred Haise would have tragically perished far from home. Instead, they lived because they were able to talk through their challenges, collaborating with the experts at NASA Mission Control. More than the successes of earlier lunar missions, it was the agency's defining moment, an illustration of why the American space program was so great.

If NASA had operated like today's U.S. health system, Apollo 13 would have ended in tragedy. The experts on the ground would have been trapped in siloed organizations, unable to share information. Even if they had managed to communicate and find a solution, they would have needed "prior authorization" from a faceless administrator before acting. By then, the capsule would have burned up on reentry. The same maze of complexity that patients struggle to navigate and that crushes the spirit of health professionals would have doomed three astronauts.

Healthcare, we have a problem.

I first grasped that truth not as a soldier or CEO, but as a child. My uncle had just returned from the Army, and our family gathered to celebrate. Driving us home, he steered through a green light when another car ran a red and slammed into us broadside. I was wedged in the front seat between my uncle and grandmother, my grandfather sitting in the back. In those days before seatbelts, the force of the crash hurled us forward.

I remember sirens, ambulances, and fire trucks. I remember my grandparents on gurneys in the ER, doctors and nurses rushing forward to care for them. What I do not remember is paperwork, insurance cards, or bureaucracy. Healers were fully engaged, urgent, and present. That was the 1960s.

The contrast with today is unavoidable. Too often, passions are buried under paperwork, metrics, and administrative demands. The system prizes compliance over compassion and process over purpose. Have we lost sight of what matters most: the instinct to heal those who need healing?

This question has defined my life. In my younger years, I was both a paratrooper and a combat medic, driven by a sense of purpose and propelled by urgency. My mission was clear: to help my friends and unit survive. On the battlefield, every decision carried life-and-death consequences. I learned quickly to act under pressure, improvise with limited resources, and never lose sight of the human being in front of me, whether friend or foe.

Years later, I traded the battlefield for the boardroom, but the mission did not change; it simply evolved. I launched and rebuilt health PR agencies, led a global turnaround, served as a private equity portfolio company CEO, and lobbied on behalf of health innovation companies. Each role sharpened my ability to navigate complexity while keeping people at the center. Today, as Chair Health and Purpose at FINN Partners, a purpose-centered global communication agency, I continue to carry the same lesson from combat medicine: communication and clarity save lives.

Perspective often emerges in unexpected places. In the first days of my marriage, I witnessed how quickly material concerns can eclipse what truly matters.

My wife and I spent our honeymoon in New York City. We didn't have much money of our own, but my in-laws treated us to a comfortable Midtown hotel, and friends generously paid for dinner at one of the city's more expensive restaurants. It was a rare taste of luxury at a time when we were starting out.

Leaving our dinner, we saw a man collapse on the sidewalk at a Fifth Avenue corner. His coins spilled across the pavement. He had a heart attack, but his words weren't about his chest pain or his life. They were about nickels and dimes: "My money, my money."

My wife knelt to gather the scattered change while I leaned into my EMT training, calling for an ambulance and doing what I could until help arrived. As the paramedics lifted him onto the stretcher, he clutched the broom he used to make a meager living. My wife placed the coins back in his hands.

In the confusion, her gold bracelet, a gift from a college friend, slipped from her wrist and disappeared. We knew the bracelet had value. However, at that moment, it was dwarfed by the man's desperate fear of losing his day's collection of coins even as his life was in jeopardy.

Standing on Fifth Avenue that night, the contrast could not have been sharper. Our hotel room, fine dinner, and bracelet all paled next to the image of a man valuing nickels and dimes more than his own survival. Sadly, that is the metaphor for our health system today, balancing life against cost. Healers are entangled in the currency of the moment rather than the urgency of preserving life.

Incidentally, the movie we had watched earlier that evening was Arthur, starring Dudley Moore as a millionaire who gave up his fortune for love. It was directed by Steve Gordon, who, coincidentally, died of a heart attack shortly after its release. The irony was striking: a story about trading wealth for what truly matters, followed by our own real-life encounter on the streets of New York that same night.

I still feel the impact of that encounter to this day. While we were grateful to have helped the man in crisis, he helped us more in many ways by offering an enduring perspective. Whether coins or jewelry, material possessions lose all value when life itself is at stake. Public retellings of Steve Jobs's final reflections point to a lesson many recognize at life's edge: the icons of success hold little power. In illness, titles and possessions recede, and what remains is an undeniable truth: life itself is the only currency that matters.

The health system must reclaim that perspective if it is to be successful and sustainable. The goal is not only to maintain health and save lives but also to recognize that profit flows from purpose. Yet too often, we see the balance reversed. Rather than holding purpose and profit in partnership, one "P," profit, is allowed to overshadow the other. When profit eclipses purpose, the system loses its way.

Executives must ask, "Am I working to benefit my customer, the patient? Am I including people in the process? Am I listening to the patients' voices? Do the environment and culture I provide help my people do their best work? Am I approving the best policies and programs that materially improve people's lives?"

We may fall short in our efforts, but we are on the right track if we work to improve care and people's lives. Refusing to consider what is at stake is a true failure. All the innovation, all the money, and all the tools we are developing will never help us reach our greatest potential if we don't return to the notion of why we are doing this in the first place.

How do we work better together, collaborating more like the experts in NASA Mission Control? We in the health system must ask ourselves whether we truly value our connections with one another. Do we recognize the contributions of patient advocacy organizations? Do we fully appreciate the relationships we have with physicians and nurses? Do we value our partnerships with payers and policymakers? Do we listen to the researchers and innovators whose breakthroughs shape the future of medicine? If we fail to honor and strengthen these relationships, we are not doing our best work.

We can do better. The fact that payers are often perceived as the enemy, as critics charge that insurers habitually delay, deny, and defend, reveals how undervalued they feel and highlights the opportunity for improvement. Consumers deeply value the medicines and devices that save their lives; shouldn't they also value the companies and researchers that bring those innovations forward? Our challenge is to stop seeing each other as adversaries and start acting as a team, united around the patient's interest.

I invite health leaders to answer a higher calling. The potential is within reach: to build sustainable, responsible businesses that deliver greater impact and, therefore, greater value. Great ideas do more than make brands visible; they make brands valuable because they improve lives.

Though the experience of too many suggests that the system values itself more than the patient, the truth is that the system has no malice. No one wakes up intending to make life harder for patients. People are trained to do their jobs, and most do them well. However, their work often serves their institution first. In hospitals, staff are judged by loyalty to their system. Policymakers are measured by party wins. Pharma leaders are evaluated by shareholder return. In that fragmented picture, where does the patient fit?

Perception reflects a painful reality. Too often, the health system has become its own customer. I am not suggesting we ignore the business side, only that we redirect equal energy toward people. The central question must be: if we care for the sustainability of our institutions, are we caring equally for the lives of patients?

We face this complexity at every moment. We cannot escape the duality of economics and patient care. The system and the patient are symbiotic. Success for one must mean success for the other.

Imagine if leaders declared, "Our legacy will be that we served people. We made medicine more accessible. We preserved the lives of parents so they could care for their children." Imagine if payers, product innovators, and policymakers said, "We will tackle heart disease and rare disease together. We will make care more accessible, reimbursement easier, and prevention a shared priority." If we could unite around even one non-communicable disease, we would unlock progress against diabetes, obesity, and other illnesses.

We often complain about the health system, and with good reason. However, this book is not about adding one more voice to the chorus of criticism. It is about how we begin to look beyond the problems, look into the mirror, and recognize that each of us has a role in healing the system. Change begins when we stop treating healthcare as someone else's responsibility and start seeing it as a national and personal commitment. Only then can we begin to build a system worthy of the people it serves.

This is our challenge and our opportunity. It is not revolutionary. It is simple. Progress begins with communication, collaboration, and the humility to improve together.

Perfection is a dream. Progress is possible. In fact, progress is enough because it changes lives. It is this ethos that frames the chapters ahead, as I explore how leaders, innovators, and communities can rally around improvement as the path to healing our fragmented health system.

Yes, healthcare, we have a problem. However, if we act urgently to collaborate with empathy, the steps we take together can lead to enduring solutions.

Chapter 1

THE PERSONAL JOURNEY: WHY THE HEALTH SYSTEM IS A FORCE FOR GOOD

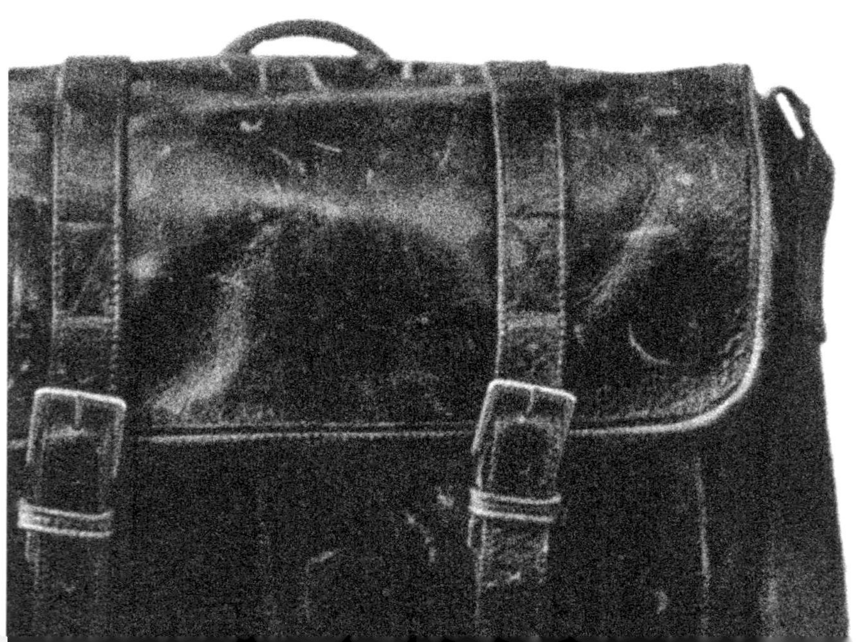

HEALTH is both a business and a mission.

Let's flip that notion for a moment. When you see the health system first as a mission, it still demands structure and resources. It requires equipment and medicines, investment in innovation, training and educating people, and making smart, sometimes difficult, choices where need is greatest. The mission and the business are inseparable. So why is the mission so often sidelined?

The answer becomes clear when you look at communities themselves. A mission without business discipline is only aspiration. If you serve neighborhoods near factories or foundries, respiratory disease or diabetes may be disproportionately common.

Research indicates that people residing near industrial facilities are at a significantly higher risk of developing respiratory illnesses. A 2020 ecological analysis in the European Journal of Environment & Public Health found that communities exposed to heavier industrial emissions experienced a significant increase in asthma prevalence. Living in a polluted environment is not merely an inconvenience; it exacts a measurable toll on the lungs and, ultimately, on one's life.

Serving those populations well requires more than compassion. It demands a tailored approach to planning, strategy, economics, and systems. This is where the business side of health can work in service of the mission.

Yet we cannot forget that all that structure is meant to support people: People who sit in hospital hallways and partitioned ER bays. People sitting nervously in physician waiting rooms, and those whose access to care depends on the continuation of telehealth policies and legislative extensions that make remote visits possible.

I often think of an episode from the classic British series Yes, Minister. In Season 2, Episode 1, the minister tours a hospital that is pristine, quiet, spotless, and orderly. Something feels off.

“Where are the patients?” he asks.

“We don’t have patients here, Minister.”

“How many work here?”

“Four hundred, Minister.”

The director explains, in earnest, how the building required guards, then a custodial crew, then a cafeteria, then HR, then administrators. The minister finally explodes, “Get patients in here next week or I’m closing the hospital!”

The director protests, “But Minister, this is an award-winning hospital.”

“Award-winning for what?”

“It’s the most hygienic hospital in the United Kingdom.”

It is absurd and uncomfortably familiar. Sometimes the business of health detaches from care. Health systems often prioritize sustainability over patient experience. People wait without clarity, repeat their histories at every visit, and feel processed. This is where mission must re-enter: to make sure people never feel like widgets in a machine.

Hospitality in a Hospital

A recent experience stayed with me. I had an exam at a large hospital. Before the appointment, the head of nursing, not a scheduler, called me personally. She confirmed the time, fasting and hydration instructions, and even asked if I had anxiety about the machine. She cared about my emotional state.

When I arrived, someone met me at the door. “Mr. Bashe?”

“Yes.”

“Hi, I’m Nick. I’ll escort you to the room.”

A brief delay followed. Nick apologized: “I’m so sorry, it’ll be about ten minutes while we clean the room.”

During the scan, they checked in: “Are you okay?”

Afterwards, they offered to bring me coffee. I said, “No need. Just point me.”

He replied, “It’s part of my responsibilities.”

I thought, this isn’t a hospital; it’s hospitality. On a return visit, it was the same. I felt like a person.

Later, I spoke with Dr. Alison Grann, the department head. I said, “I visit a lot of hospitals professionally. This place is different.”

She answered, “I want everyone, staff and patients, treated the way I want to be treated. I make sure my staff takes lunch and goes home on time. If extra work needs doing, the doctors and I take it on.”

At a follow-up, a nurse remembered my wife’s medical procedure from two months earlier and asked how it went.

This is not standard practice; it is personal care. It is the place where business yields to mission, and mission gives rise to meaning. Business says, “I have a schedule to keep.” Mission says, “I have a story to hear.”

The time difference might be one extra minute. Yet doctors are trained by systems that say, “See twelve patients a day.” This is the business of medicine. However, what about the moment someone hears “cancer”? A hospital may earn significant revenue from complex diagnoses, yet a physician can still be forced by the clock to deliver life-altering news and walk out. Imagine not acknowledging the shock the patient may be experiencing. Ten more minutes can change a life.

In today’s practice environment, physicians are often limited to 12- to 16-minute encounters. Studies of U.S. primary care, published in the JAMA Health Forum in

2023, reveal that average visit lengths range from 14 to 19 minutes, creating an experience that can feel more transactional than relational. Increasingly, health is something done to us, not with us.

When Technology Serves People

The "utopian" experience is rare, but not unheard of. Technology can help. At NYU Langone, a major academic medical center in New York City, I checked in on an iPad and a nurse arrived within a minute. The device did more than register me; it activated the care system. Handprint ID now recalls records and alerts the care team in real time. This is an example of technology supporting both the business and the mission.

When technology serves only business, patients think, "When will they get to me?" I've waited 90 minutes for an appointment, which tells patients their time isn't valued.

As a customer of this system, I don't expect perfection. I want to feel the system cares about me. I want empathy to stand alongside efficiency. The business side matters, but it must be shaped and softened by the mission. For too long, we have leaned on business without enough focus on mission. It's time to rebalance.

A Life of Observation

As a rabbi, I am invited into people's most vulnerable moments. I witness their pain when a loved one is

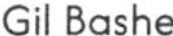

gravely ill or dying, and their joy when a life has been well lived. I see bonds between families and caregivers. I'm moved when a physician asks to speak at a funeral, and I notice when they are absent. In these moments, medicine's clinical and emotional dimensions reveal themselves most clearly.

Over the years, people have turned to me for guidance: "I've just been diagnosed. Who should I see? Who do you trust?" I connect them to physicians who are both top-tier clinicians and true healers. Then I stay involved, following up with patients, doctors, and families. I walk with them through the journey.

I think of physicians like Dr. Allyson Ocean at Weill Cornell, a gastrointestinal oncologist who specializes in treating pancreatic cancer. Her patients know the odds. Many see in her not just brilliance, but an open heart and an emotional pillar in a difficult chapter. Dr. Ocean has empowered patients by creating Let's Win Pancreatic Cancer, a crowdsourcing network, so people won't have to face the journey alone.

I spend time with doctors like her, leaders who lead from the heart. I also serve on boards across the ecosystem: I was a regional chair of the American Heart Association, I sit on the boards of the American Diabetes Association and the Marfan Foundation, and I advise Let's Win Pancreatic Cancer. These roles immerse me in the realities of chronic and life-threatening illness.

Through it all, I've come to a simple truth: care has a business side, but the mission is about relationships.

Relationships keep me grounded in both faith and medicine. They are also what turn skilled providers into exceptional healers.

This perspective is personal, too. My late father-in-law, Dr. Burt Giges, was a formative influence in the field. First in his class at the NYU School of Medicine, he later worked in infectious disease at Walter Reed and Rockefeller University before becoming a leader in psychiatry and sports psychology. At 94, he continued to see patients. He lived and breathed patient care. For decades, I sat across a kitchen table from a man devoted to doing right by others.

My wife is a psychologist, bound by confidentiality but open about the emotional experience and privilege of helping people change. Emotional insight is a gem that illuminates the journey.

Our daughter lives with a rare disease. Nearly every week brings a new appointment or decision. I've seen how the system responds—or doesn't. As a licensed social worker and award-winning author, she writes about characters with disabilities. Her perseverance is a teacher.

I also think of my grandmother, a survivor who helped raise me, and of my parents. My mother died of uterine cancer, or more precisely, of fear. She avoided seeking medical help for her prolonged bleeding until it was too late. I begged her, "Mom, see an OB-GYN now." My father, already ill with Parkinson's disease, died of Crohn's—or perhaps of treatment that focused on the disease to the exclusion of him. This distinction matters. Both my parents died of non-communicable, treatable illnesses, and in both cases, fear of the diagnosis and distrust of the system played a role.

That fear was compounded by the system's own failures. As my mother lay dying, I discovered that an OB-GYN at a major academic medical center had identified a new tumor just a week before her death. Yet the physician delayed notifying her oncologist—both practicing in the same hospital—until clinical notes could be typed up and faxed. The oncologist, unaware of the deadly threat, continued treating as if the tumor didn't exist. Standing at her bedside, I asked both distinguished physicians what they had learned. Their unison reply was haunting: "We should have communicated with each other immediately."

Professionally, these experiences are part of my internal inventory. I also conduct research for broader perspective. In May 1995, at the dawn of the World Wide Web, I published a study in Product Management Today that showed people with chronic illnesses often feel a stronger connection to others with the same condition than to their healthy neighbors. Illness reshapes identity and builds bonds that cut across race, geography, and class.

Too often, the system fails to adapt to meet those needs. Consider our daughter. She needed a capsule endoscopy (the so-called "smart pill"), a safe, established, less invasive option used by hundreds of thousands. The insurer called it "experimental" despite the decades of research and insisted on endoscopy, colonoscopy, and a gastric emptying test. Three procedures instead of one. We paid out of pocket; the pill identified slow motility tied to her rare disease. Why default to what's harder on the patient when the better solution is cheaper and proven? Where is the empathy?

These situations are not abstract; they play out in real lives every day, in small but anxiety-filled moments when people in distress find themselves waiting, sometimes for hours, not only for care but to be believed.

The words of a caregiver on Reddit's r/AskDocs forum caught my eye, describing how his 37-year-old partner spent more than ten hours in an ER acute waiting area experiencing what was ultimately diagnosed as a deadly pulmonary embolism. Her racing heart and growing anxiety were repeatedly reported, yet the couple felt dismissed as if youth made the symptoms less pressing. Only after a long-awaited scan revealed blood clots did the care team shift from curt to attentive. The caregiver shared the ordeal crystallized a quiet terror shared by many patients and families in similar situations: that someone you love can suffer in plain sight while waiting to be believed.

Constraints are real. But people can be treated like human beings, not transactions.

Take, for example, a woman with a questionable mammogram. What follows? Women are often left carrying both the anxiety of a suspicious result and the added burden of advocating for themselves within the system. For those with dense breast tissue, the path becomes even more fragmented: the mammogram on one day, the ultrasound on another, each requiring time away from work or family and extending the emotional strain. If the images raise further concern, she must find a physician to perform the biopsy and hope that office accepts her insurance, receives her imaging records and fits her into a crowded schedule.

Then comes the longest stretch: waiting a week or more for pathology results. During those days of silence, when the system has no mechanism to calm anxieties, uncertainty becomes its own form of suffering. The clinical steps of detection and diagnosis are well understood; the human experience of navigating them, especially for women who face delays, access barriers, and logistical hurdles, is not. These unseen gaps reveal the emotional weight of fragmented care.

Recently, we received a two-page denial letter with no reason or details provided. My wife asked what I thought. I said, “I have no idea.” She called the company. They didn’t either. Language no one understands—who benefits from that? Imagine any other service business run that way. How long would it last?

I am a sponge for stories. Everyone in the system brings their psychological history, and the system often overlooks it. Pain is not just physical. Emotional hurt doesn’t show up on an MRI. It’s real. Our health system rarely recognizes that dimension.

“Doctor, I don’t think you’re listening.” The truthful answer might be, “I really want to, but I don’t have time.” Is that the best we can do?

The Language of Empathy

Medical training includes physiology, pharmacology, and procedures, but little on patient experience. Yet the core mission of being a physician is dealing with people.

Some specialties reduce interaction by design. In radiology, the technician is visible; the radiologist is behind a glass partition. In surgery, you may meet the surgeon twice, briefly, before and after. For the patient, that "transaction" is everything.

The system is not structured to prioritize human connection. Doctors are trained to operate, diagnose, and prescribe. Listening and connecting are assumed—not taught, measured, or rewarded. As the saying goes, you respect what you inspect. If empathy isn't inspected, don't expect it to thrive.

So what makes a great doctor? Surgical precision matters. But so does this—when our daughter needed a rare abdominal surgery, we traveled to Santa Monica to see Dr. Danny Shouhed, a gifted robotic surgeon. What made him unforgettable wasn't just the successful precision operation. While we waited, he phoned: "Where are you?"

"The cafeteria."

"I'll come down." He arrived with scans, walked us through the plan, answered every question, and laid out next steps. He didn't just perform surgery; he showed up for two anxious parents, a person first, doctor second. He even gave us his personal cell phone number.

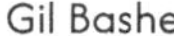

These small acts of kindness define greatness: remembering that behind every scan and chart is a human being.

We talk about empathy and compassion but rarely build them into the system. We ask nurses to be gracious in the face of pain, but don't give them the time or support to care. Twelve-hour shifts, unit floating, constant gaps. Burnout is predictable.

We know why they burn out. We haven't decided it's important enough to fix.

How many bedside nurses in their fifties still want to be there? Many are exhausted and counting the days. Can we blame them? We haven't made the job sustainable or human.

Meanwhile, we invest heavily in innovation. We are not lacking in ideas or tools, but we are lacking in connection and purpose.

What the Battlefield Taught Me

Recently, in May 2025, the remains of a soldier missing for decades were finally returned to his family. I had fought in that same battle decades earlier. The moment reminded me how some experiences never truly fade; they shape how we carry ourselves long after. Healthcare is no different. A diagnosis, a kind gesture, or a failure of empathy leaves an imprint that lingers for years. These moments, whether lived by patients, families, or providers, become the compass that keeps us oriented toward purpose and humanity in every decision we make.

Battle teaches what most try to avoid: that life is fragile, temporary, and unpredictable. You see things you can't unsee. In the middle of it, your job is to function, to help, to hold the line—and to keep your humanity. Lose that, and you lose more than a battle.

I watched vehicles vanish in balls of flame. As a soldier and paramedic, I realized the only thing I could truly hold onto was humanity and my purpose. I had to save lives fast, without losing the part of me that felt. Caring for a wounded enemy soldier was an act of defiance against chaos; it was my way of saying, "If I were on the other side, I'd pray someone would help me."

I'm not describing heroism. I was terrified. I wanted to live, like everyone else. Some moments don't fade; they grow sharper. They remind you what you survived and who you became.

Every healer knows that urgency. The work doesn't wash off.

At some point, we will all be sick, frightened, and vulnerable. When that day comes, we will want someone to bring not just skill but presence. All that they have.

Why am I still so passionate? In my professional life, I am a health communicator who has experienced this profession from both sides of the table: from clinical papers and product launches, to the edge and the abyss. Like the healer at day's end, it never fully washes off.

There's no war in my daily life now, but there is suffering, despair, and people praying for a lifeline. Doctors, innovation, and communication can help. So I give it everything I've got, every time.

Healing doesn't have a native language. It is presence, time, and touch. It's the way you speak to a person, the way you examine them, the way you treat not just an illness but a life.

On the battlefield, I triaged a soldier whose arm was attached by skin and whose femur was shattered by shrapnel. There was blood loss, shock, the question of salvage, and the clock. We stabilized, triaged, and evacuated as a team. That is medicine at its core.

Some memories return in flashes: armored cars hit ahead of me; the thought that their mothers wanted their children to live just as much as my mother wanted me to live. In the conventional battlefields of my youth, war was a machine in which people on both sides did their duty, hoping to return home alive. Today, the landscape is more complex. Some combatants, shaped by extremist indoctrination, may even embrace death as part of their mission. Yet even amid these stark differences, the fundamental truth remains: most people, in most wars, still yearn for life and for the chance to return safely to the families who wait for them.

My pride is not in being fearless. It is in staying human. That is the open-door invitation in medicine: to be human, especially when things look terrible.

The Doctor's Black Bag

Until recently, the pace of innovation we see today didn't exist. Gene therapy, biotech, and digital tools were once unimaginable but are now routine. Robotic surgery is no longer science fiction. Many mainstay cholesterol drugs emerged in the 1990s and early 2000s. Breakthrough immunotherapies, such as PD-1 inhibitors for cancer, are products of the last decade.

Specialization has deepened, too. "Cardiologist" once covered the whole heart. Now we have electrophysiologists, interventional cardiologists, and cardiothoracic surgeons. Gastroenterology has become increasingly specialized, with a focus on ever-narrower areas. This sharpens expertise but introduces problems. Specialists may miss how one system affects another. Additionally, we tend to adopt a symptomatic approach, treating the visible symptoms without inquiring about underlying causes.

My father-in-law taught me to start with why. Don't reflexively prescribe for reflux; ask if it's diet, weight, physiology, or something masquerading as GERD. Great physicians question the root cause.

Today, we're highly symptomatic in treatment analogues. Consider asthma. Providers often say, "Here's an inhaler," without asking why episodes spike. Maybe it's heat exposure without air conditioning. Maybe it's housing. Maybe food insecurity explains a child's GI complaint or ADHD-like behavior.

Are we giving healers the bandwidth to find out? Increasingly, no.

In earlier decades, primary care physicians held a fuller role. They knew your story. They asked about your family. They were in your community, visible at the diner or place of worship. They didn't just refer. They reasoned with you about why.

As specialization and consolidation have grown, personal connections have become increasingly thin. Walk-in clinics can be convenient, but they are often transactional. “My shoulder hurts.” The X-ray looks fine. “Here’s a pain med.” The shoulder pain may be the messenger, not the message.

I grew up when physicians knew their patients, and patients knew their physicians. Our pediatrician, Dr. Brody, even made house calls, black bag in hand, and brought a toy when I was sick. Years later, while cleaning my in-laws’ home after my father-in-law's death, I found his black leather bag. It stirred memories of both men and the people-first ethos they carried.

My relationship with medicine shifted again when I became an emergency care provider in the military. Medics are called “Doc.” I wasn’t a doctor, but in the middle of nowhere, for the people entrusted to me, I was the closest thing. I ran infusions, gave injectables, and performed minor procedures. I rotated through ER, surgery, GI, and grand rounds. These were deep relationships—different from Dr. Brody’s, but still deeply human. Health was interconnected: both clinical and personal.

What’s Going Wrong

At FINN Partners, culture is paramount. If a client behaves abusively, we address it. If it continues, we walk away. We aspire to be the “best place to work,” and that requires protecting our people. We value both people and productivity. It’s not one or the other.

This respect is often missing in the health system. Burnout among physicians and nurses is no longer whispered about; it is a well-documented reality across the healthcare ecosystem, a fact underscored by the American Medical Association, which notes that burnout affects every specialty and practice setting. It's not just the workload; it's the environment: legal pressure in the event of a medical error, stress if you don't see enough patients, and schedules that leave little time for thoughtful care. We need to consider how economics and workflow impact the emotional well-being of health professionals and their effect on patient care.

Most people enter the field of medicine because they are drawn to the healing profession. We do not nurture that desire or reward it. On the administrative side, leaders rightly worry about economic viability; hospital margins are thin. Payer margins are different; many are highly profitable within larger corporations. Throughput becomes the metric. Staff experience becomes a footnote.

Some systems run by physicians streamline non-clinical costs and reinvest in frontline staff. When they do, both the caregiver and the patient experience improvement.

Training matters, too. Electronic medical records are cumbersome. When my 97-year-old father-in-law spent his final 13 days in an excellent New York Metro hospital, a nurse asked me something I knew was already recorded in his EMR. I said so. She replied, "I don't have time to read the EMR." She had twelve new patients. He had a new nurse almost daily. That is not sustainable.

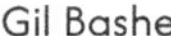

Technology can help. Imagine AI tools summarizing a patient's record at shift start: What matters for the next twelve hours? Technology should work for caregivers and people, not just for legal protection.

We can be more profitable and more human-centered when caregivers are enabled to be full allies in a person's well-being. Medicine is not managing cholesterol or gallbladders; it is helping whole people.

Many chronic conditions, like type 2 diabetes, can improve with lifestyle change. Colleagues have put diabetes into remission through weight loss, exercise, and specialized diets. Yet reimbursement rarely covers what works: sustained nutrition counseling, physical activity support, and social determinants that create obstacles to healing. Physicians are not enabled to prescribe the team a patient needs.

We tie our hands by prioritizing cost and compliance over impact. I've seen payers where one representative says yes, and another says no to the same question. Clinical decisions are sometimes made by individuals outside the relevant specialty. That is a breakdown on top of a breakdown.

We need to rethink the cost of saying "no." What are the emotional, physical, and long-term financial impacts? Does the person feel supported or abandoned?

Too often, no one has your back unless you know how to work the system. Most doctors don't want their patients to suffer or face obstacles in obtaining the necessary care. They want to help.

I recall when a widely respected physician, John Rowe, MD, a leader in public health and later the President of Mount Sinai, eventually led the health insurance giant Aetna. He simplified the prior authorization process after discovering that it cost more to process the paperwork than to provide the service itself. The company enjoyed a long period of profitability. It is possible to draw from playbooks that work, aligning people and profit.

We need to step back and assess everyone's experience: people, providers, and leaders. It isn't mission or business. The mission is the business of care delivery. People in the trenches, including doctors, nurses, technicians, and sanitation staff, care deeply about people. People in the ivory tower often fail to recognize reality.

My grounding came as a paramedic. After my military service, I volunteered with an urban ambulance squad. The most important tool wasn't my bag; it was the ability to sit, listen, and reassure—to see the person in front of me.

Once on vacation, during a transatlantic flight, turbulence hit hard. The call went out: "Any medical personnel on board?" Silence. The call repeated. My wife nudged me, and I stepped forward. A man had fainted and was mortified—he had lost bladder control. I quickly ran cognitive checks: name, date, and then the current U.S. president. He passed the usual checks. Likely dehydration, perhaps worsened by an in-flight drink. I reassured him, suggested fluids, and urged him to see a doctor after landing.

A neurologist sitting two rows back later said, "I would have done exactly that." But he hadn't moved.

The 30,000-foot exchange in the air reflects a deeper problem, not just in medicine but in leadership across fields. We hesitate. We freeze. Paperwork, liability, and fear pile up. Action stalls. Yet when someone is suffering, we have a duty to step in. This call to act belongs not only to clinicians but to business leaders, policymakers, and communicators.

I carry a stethoscope when I travel, along with a small KardiaMobile, a medical-grade device that detects irregular heartbeats, also known as arrhythmias. Not because I expect to save lives daily, but because the person before me is a person—not a symptom, not a file. Human, anxious, deserving of care.

In health communication, I channel that empathy. A company's message should not only inform but also inspire action and well-being. Great communication from companies, innovators, physicians, and nurses elevates awareness and motivates engagement.

This is my business mission: to help people reduce their health burden and access the best that innovation has to offer.

The bottom line: the business of medicine requires two balance sheets. One measures dollars and cents. The other measures people: health, satisfaction, trust, and the well-being of the professionals who provide care. Ignore either, and the system collapses. If innovation or delivery cannot sustain itself, if inner-city hospitals cannot cover salaries and keep the lights on, care breaks down.

When people are treated as if they don't matter, they disengage, avoid going to the doctor, delay care, become sicker, and ultimately incur higher costs. This is not only a matter of morality; it is also simple economics.

Equally vital are time and respect for health professionals. Squeezing every minute out of physicians, nurses, and allied teams leads to burnout, turnover, and declining quality. When clinicians are exhausted and unsupported, the human connection erodes and no technology or billing efficiency can replace it.

We will create an effective, efficient, and empathetic system only when humanity shares equal weight with economics and when professionals have the time and permission to do their best work.

In 2000, I wrote an article for Pharmaceutical Executive about the importance of emotion as a brand integrator. At that time, marketers began to realize that attributes and features were not enough to differentiate their products; it was the emotional connection that made a brand truly resonate with its community. Twenty-five years later, our health system is at a similar crossroads. We are layering information and technology on shaky foundations, hoping they will hold. Just as with brands, the real breakthrough will not come from adding more features. It will come when we recognize that empathy and connection between those who deliver care and those who receive it are foundational integrators of health.

Chapter 2

A FRAGMENTED SYSTEM: PITTING PROFIT AGAINST CARE

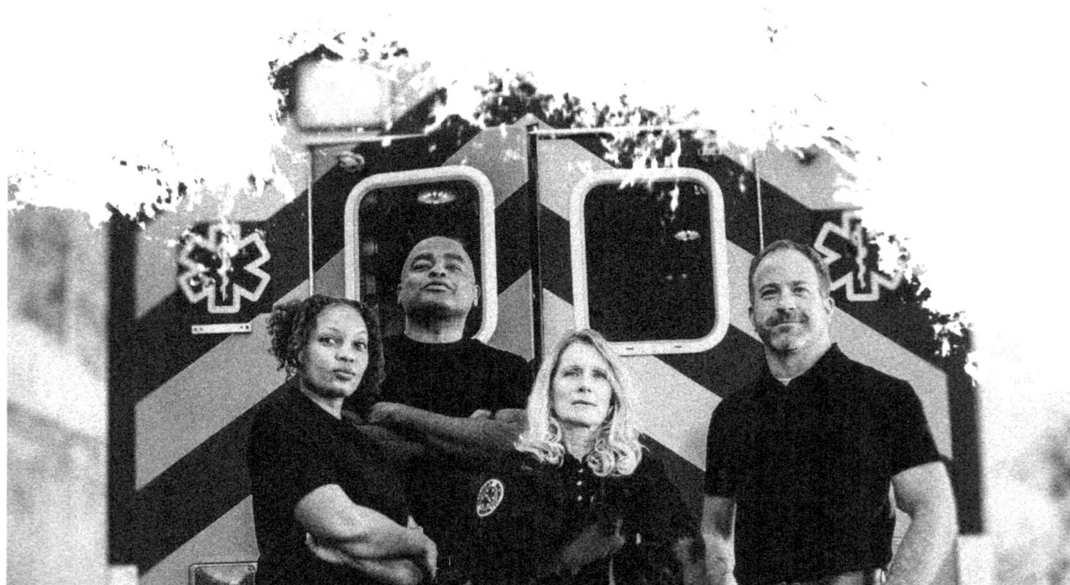

IN December 2024, O'Dwyer's PR magazine invited me to write a piece about the assassination of Brian Thompson. Thompson was an executive at UnitedHealthcare, but it could just as easily have been someone from any other health insurance organization.

Most likely, the unacceptable public reaction—ranging from "Who's next?" to "He deserved it"—would have been the same. UnitedHealthcare's official condolence posts were met with derision; the bereavement message on Facebook reportedly drew tens of thousands of "laughing" reactions.

Thompson's assassination was deeply tragic, made even more disturbing by public insensitivity that treated murder as protest and vigilantism as justice.

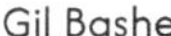

In my article, I discussed what industry should do moving forward: prioritize the experience of the people the system intends to serve.

Putting patient experience first is not a standard goal in the industry. It means recognizing that people who are ill are worried, scared, sometimes in denial, and often clueless about the process. How can we improve their experience? How can we design the system to work effectively for the customer?

I am not purposely incognito when in a hospital, but it's safe to say people do not realize I'm also curating experiences and a writer who focuses on the health business. People see me as a patient or a family member of a patient, not someone who is constantly observing. In truth, I approach every interaction as a case study, observing how the health system either supports or fails the people it is meant to serve.

I recently had an extraordinary experience at a hospital. Forget valet parking; people visiting for treatment could park right at the center's door. I was met at the door and treated as a guest. I was utterly amazed. I thought, "Wow, what an easy experience."

At other hospitals, I continually circle massive parking lots, seeking an empty spot. To an extent, that is understandable, in the same way it is in the parking lot of a shopping center. However, people tend to be more worried when visiting a hospital than when shopping. They are more anxious about arriving on time and about the procedure they or their loved one will be undergoing.

It is not an accident that the health system's breakdown is partly caused by executives' failure to prioritize customer experience, which should be central to their mission.

Despite my wife's and my experience within the health business, the legal jargon in an insurance carrier's letter can still be bewildering. We often find ourselves calling to ask, in plain English, what the company actually needs from us. That is not a customer-centered approach; it is simply the industry norm. Insurers have the ability and resources to communicate more clearly, yet too often they choose not to. When insurers communicate clearly, people feel less overwhelmed and are more able to focus on getting care, rather than decoding paperwork.

When I receive a call from my health insurance company saying they have assigned a nurse to assist me, I do not assume they have assigned a nurse to help me. Instead, I assume they have assigned a nurse to oversee my doctor's work. In other words, I assume the insurance company's interests are not aligned with my doctor's. Many insurance companies' options no longer even allow patients to choose their doctors beyond their primary care provider. The patient-doctor relationship, which has been established over time, is marginalized.

The health system has five pillars. The five "Ps" are patients, payers (health insurance companies), policymakers, product innovators, and providers (healthcare professionals).

These pillars support the edifice of care and should be mutually supportive; however, the system's interests are so out of alignment that the pillars often operate almost independently of each other, seeming to exist in parallel universes. They do not support one another and fail to place the patient at the center of their activities. Instead, they align around creating checks and balances for themselves. It's no wonder patients do not trust the system.

This is where the breakdown lies.

A System Disconnected

Doctors and other health system workers operate within their respective disciplines to address patient needs. They are neither inherently collaborative nor uncollaborative.

A doctor's most pressing concern is when, and even whether, the payer will approve. In my experience, many doctors want to, or are required to, proceed with diagnostic tests or treatment. Instead, they are obligated to spend an hour on the phone with the patient's health insurance company trying to convince them that a particular medical treatment is necessary.

Of course, health insurance companies can be justified in denying a request if they have deemed a medical procedure clinically unnecessary. Keep in mind, insurers' employees do not work for free. In a way, they are saying, "Look, it's not that we don't want you to have what you need. We feel what you're already getting will be sufficient, but if it isn't, then of course we'll revisit our decision."

If an insurance carrier chooses not to cover a medical cost, the patient is left holding the bag. Those with more means may occasionally choose to see a provider and pay for the visit. However, tests and procedures are out of reach for most without insurance. Increasingly, even certain procedures may be out of reach for all but the extraordinarily wealthy.

Consider 17-year-old Nataline Sarkisyan, whose doctors recommended a liver transplant that her insurer denied as "experimental." After public outcry, the insurer reversed its decision, but she died within hours of the approval. Her story illustrates how delays and denials can render lifesaving care inaccessible to those without extraordinary means.

Where do the patient's experience, the doctor's expertise, and the best clinical evidence fit into that conversation? A successful health outcome largely depends on whether the doctor or provider effectively advocates for their patient. Remember, the doctor must explain the company's decision to the patient, who is treated like a child in this transactional conversation.

In this country, we do not have a health system; we have a sick care system. A true health system would focus on prevention and early intervention. According to Federal data from the Centers for Medicare & Medicaid Services (CMS) and analyses by the Trust for America's Health, only about 2.5 to three percent of U.S. health spending goes to public health and prevention, while the remaining 97 percent is spent on treating diseases after they have appeared. Instead of helping people stay well, the system waits until they are ill, leaving patients to navigate a maze of appointments, authorizations, and bills when it is often too late.

This is not a book about the millions who already lack access to basic care, though their struggle should weigh heavily on us. It is about a system that falls short even for those who manage to do everything right. For families living paycheck to paycheck, the first step is securing insurance that covers both preventive and acute care. Then comes the task of finding a provider who accepts that coverage, such as Medicaid, and offers the necessary services.

Yet, the obstacles don't end there. Patients must carve out time from work or childcare to make the appointment, often at clinics where waits stretch for hours. Even with discounted fees, affordability remains a barrier. Specialists usually have long wait times, and primary care offices are frequently full. For many, the only remaining option is urgent care, which comes with a $50 copay that can feel overwhelming for families already struggling to make ends meet. If the system fails those who fight hardest to use it, how can we pretend it is built for anyone?

Sickness is scary. No one wants to be sick. However, in many cases, people have to be encouraged or invited to seek treatment. Few insurance companies in the U.S. call when you are overdue for your colonoscopy, prostate exam, primary physician check, or pap smear. Illness would still exist if the system were more proactive, but it would be detected earlier. This would most likely lead to a better outcome.

When I was a child, I remember watching countless children, predominantly people of color, cross the street to my father's gas station, where he had candy and soda machines to make a little extra revenue. Often, they would buy a Coca-Cola and a candy bar for breakfast. Back then, someone with limited buying power could buy breakfast for 50 cents.

Fast food has long offered Americans convenience at the expense of nutrition, contributing quietly but powerfully to rising rates of chronic disease. Today, however, we are starting to see change. More chains are recognizing their responsibility in shaping public health and expanding healthier options. It reflects a growing responsible-business mindset: when companies widen access to nutritious choices, they play a concrete role in supporting a healthier nation.

Someone who skips lunch and walks by a café at three o'clock will most likely opt for a cheaper, yet tastier option, such as a piece of cake, a donut, or a cookie, rather than a more expensive option like a salad with avocado toast and protein. In studies, low-income households purchase fewer fruits and vegetables and more sugar-sweetened beverages compared with higher-income households, even when living in the same city. If they do choose the more expensive option, it's often only because they are fortunate enough to afford it.

The cherry on top is that this unhealthy food is highly palatable. Thus, by making unhealthy food cheaper, our society essentially perpetuates diabetes, obesity, and heart disease—no wonder they're so prevalent.

The U.S. obesity crisis continues to widen, with more than 40 percent of adults and nearly 20 percent of children and teens affected; figures drawn from the CDC's 2024 surveillance reports, which track obesity trends across the country.

Nearly one in ten Americans now live with severe obesity, according to CDC 2023–2024 data, yet fewer than two percent of eligible patients receive anti-obesity medications, as shown in recent analyses from the American Medical Association. This gap largely reflects economic constraints, and even when people want help, access remains limited. Currently, approximately 100 board-certified obesity specialists practice in the United States, making expert guidance exceptionally difficult to obtain. Barriers to treatment are not simply medical; they are structural.

Federal government-funded studies from 2021 and 2022 indicate that lower-income families often prioritize what they can afford over what is most nutritious. As far back as 2013, analysis found that better-quality diets cost more, a reality that is expected and strains families already struggling to make ends meet. Policymakers talk about obesity but rarely address how closely poverty and illness are linked. Until they do, we will continue to treat symptoms rather than addressing the underlying conditions that contribute to illness and its associated costs.

Increased engagement from the health system could save lives and lower costs by treating obesity for what it is: a complex medical condition that deserves expert attention. Many people live with genetic, metabolic, or medication-related factors that cannot be solved with generic advice, yet only a small fraction of insurance plans cover access to board-certified obesity specialists. Medicare coverage is minimal. Most commercial insurers exclude structured, specialist-guided care altogether. The result is predictable: patients are left without the personalized assessment their condition requires. This is a system gap, not a personal failing.

So people do what people always do: they find a way. Many now turn to direct-to-patient services, including telehealth platforms that provide compounded GLP-1 medications through licensed pharmacies. Some individuals choose these options because insurance does not cover the FDA-approved therapies. Others choose them because they are simply easier to access than traditional pathways. In a system this hard to navigate, convenience becomes its own form of compassion. When patients must look outside the system for the care they need, it's a sign that the system, not the individual, must change.

This gap persists even though obesity drives an estimated $173 billion in annual medical spending in the United States, according to CDC data, largely through downstream costs from diabetes, heart disease, and cancer. We understand the cost of avoidance and know what works. The barrier is a system that has yet to prioritize the medical and mental well-being of the people most affected. Until we make proven support accessible, we cannot expect to see changes in outcomes.

When we fail to prioritize both body and mind, we force millions of people to navigate a medical condition with psychological, financial, and emotional tolls that no one can be expected to carry alone. It is as though we have withdrawn from the health system's mandate to protect people from this epidemic, choosing instead to underwrite the far greater expense of advanced disease. In effect, society subsidizes the sickness industry. Our approach is backward.

Medicaid is a safety net for people with financial constraints in the U.S. However, policymakers have implemented an 80-hour work month requirement for eligibility, which is set to take effect in January 2027. This will instantly make millions of people ineligible. What if parents who must work for Medicaid eligibility can't afford childcare? What about people with medical conditions that prevent steady work? The irony is that working these hours could disqualify those same people from getting disability income.

Many times, people stay home and do little to no work, not because they're unwilling, but because their children cannot be left unattended. According to Census Bureau data, around 15 percent of such parents report being unemployed specifically to care for children, and for parents of younger kids, that number rises to 35 percent. They wonder, "Who will watch my kids? The street? Will the government someday provide free daycare or after-school programming?"

Therein lies yet another problem. Where will the money for free daycare and after-school programming come from? It is as if the breakdown says, "Wait a minute. Allow me to address one population's needs while creating two more problems in the process."

The systems of European countries tend to differ from ours because the government, rather than private industries, funds their health systems. In theory, government-provided health systems could eliminate some of the issues we face in the U.S. That said, patients would still need to learn to navigate the government system and wait for care. For instance, the government may fund a knee replacement, but a patient may need to wait half a year for the surgery.

Fragmentation exists not only in the U.S. but globally. For example, the U.S. Agency for International Development (USAID) previously supported vaccination programs in low- and middle-income countries, including parts of Africa. When these efforts are halted, vaccination rates can decline, increasing the risk of localized outbreaks of diseases such as Ebola or measles. In a connected world, where millions of people travel across borders each day, gaps in vaccination anywhere pose risks everywhere. These challenges are compounded when agencies like the CDC face funding shortfalls, making coordinated tracking and response more difficult.

Charity can fill urgent gaps, but it is not a sustainable path forward. Lasting progress emerges when operational models work for both the sponsors of health innovation and the health professionals delivering care, aligning incentives around people's needs rather than temporary relief. Evidence shows that healthier populations enhance economic productivity; the World Bank estimates that as much as one-quarter of global

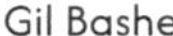

GDP growth in recent decades can be attributed to improvements in population health. When health improves, economies improve and households benefit.

This begs the critical questions: What will happen when we face another pandemic? Can it be prevented? It would most likely be less expensive to prevent it than to endure it. The breakdown persists when government and health officials are not on the same page or are in conflict.

The System Serves Itself

Each pillar of the American health system operates on its own financial "survive or thrive" objectives, rarely aligned with the others. Payers, providers, hospitals, and innovators each play by different rules, and too often, they don't even understand how the others sustain their business models. Payers may report strong profits, while many hospitals fight to keep margins above two percent.

I saw this firsthand when my daughter spent 26 hours in the ER for chronic illness complications. The hospital billed nearly $50,000. My insurer reimbursed less than $2,000, calling that the "reasonable and customary charge." The hospital had no choice but to accept it. To compensate for insurers shortchanging them, hospitals inflate their charges; in response, insurers further reduce their payments, and the cycle continues. Each side plays a money-focused game, with patients and families caught in the middle.

After that experience, I was left with two questions: How did the hospital arrive at a $50,000 bill? How did the insurer decide only $2,000 was acceptable? No one can answer. The process remains a mystery.

This is not always neglect by design, but it is the result of a fragmented culture. Each stakeholder is focused on protecting its own bottom line rather than centering its infrastructure on the consumer. The result is a system that too often forgets why it exists, to keep people healthy and return the sick to health.

Again, sickness is scary, and no one wants it. The health system understands that. Nurses become nurses, doctors become doctors, and pharmacists become pharmacists to help us get healthy. Even health insurance companies wish to prevent sickness, if only so they don't have to pay for it. On one side of the equation, the system was established to preserve your health. On the other side, the system manages the budget.

We must also consider that no one is making money if a hospital is empty. Even if the system genuinely wishes to help people, there is a built-in conflict of interest. Humans are incentivized to stay alive, while insurance companies are incentivized to stay in business.

This conflict of interest is not entirely negative. Communities need core services such as OB-GYN, cardiology, and orthopedics, but hospitals differ in their ability to provide these services effectively. We have built centers of excellence with distinct demographic strengths. The real task now is to shape every system around the human experience rather than institutional routines.

Medical expenses resulting from inadequate or unaffordable health system coverage are a primary reason for household debt in America. Many Americans lack comprehensive insurance or face high deductibles and co-pays, leaving them vulnerable to overwhelming medical debt from unexpected bills. In fact, according to Kaiser Health News' 2022 "Diagnosis: Debt" study, 41 percent of U.S. adults report carrying some form of medical debt. Even those with insurance can face substantial out-of-pocket expenses due to high deductibles, co-pays, and uncovered expenses, leading to financial strain.

Additionally, the complexity of the healthcare system, including billing practices and a lack of transparency, can make it challenging for patients to comprehend their costs and navigate the system effectively. This leads to unexpected bills and limited coverage. The absence of universal health system coverage in the U.S. exacerbates the problem, as many people are uninsured, leaving them at risk for accumulating medical debt.

A Kaiser Family Foundation "Burden of Medical Debt" in the United States 2023 survey suggests that people in the U.S. owe at least $220 billion in medical debt, with nearly 20 million adults, about one in twelve, carrying that burden. Medical debt disproportionately falls on the sickest and those least able to afford it, but its impact reaches deep into the middle class as well.

A family with a seriously ill child can quickly sink into poverty as bills pile up, even with insurance. Those with higher incomes may be able to absorb costs more easily, while lower-income families often face barriers to qualifying for assistance. Payers rarely absorb the cost, government programs offer little relief, and while Medicare can sometimes help a child with disabilities or chronic illness, approval is slow and uncertain.

The system is built not on compassion or empathy, but on policy and economics. We must add a third component to building the system: the empathetic heart upon which medicine is ultimately based.

Still, shining examples of the system working in the consumer's favor can be found. For example, the NYU Langone Health System has upheld its pledge to be patient-centered and patient-friendly. During my visits to the hospital, regardless of whom I speak to (whether a nurse or a café worker), I immediately sense the consumer-centric environment.

NYU Langone is not alone in its approach; it has joined Cleveland Clinic, Vanderbilt University Medical Center, St. Barnabas Health Network, and the Robert Wood Johnson Health Network in New Jersey. However, these organizations are the exception, not the rule. Of course, their goal is lofty and aspirational; however, that they seek to organize around patient experience should be the standard for others.

Across multiple analyses, not-for-profit health systems, such as the Mayo Clinic and Cooper, consistently rank at the higher end of the quality curve. National data link not-for-profit hospitals to lower mortality and readmission rates, higher patient satisfaction, and stronger staff morale compared with for-profit facilities. More than 20 years ago, Canadian cardiologist

Philip James Devereaux, MD, published a landmark study in the Canadian Medical Association Journal examining 26,000 hospitals and 38 million patients. His findings were striking: mortality rates were significantly lower in not-for-profit hospitals than in their for-profit counterparts.

Conversely, for-profit hospitals had poorer results, while doctors felt hassled and patients felt neglected.

That's not to say hospital systems should all be not-for-profit. It is an opportunity for the leadership of for-profit hospitals to embrace a new perspective. They must say, "Our institution exists not only for the sake of the institution, but primarily for the people we serve and a setting for those seeking to heal. These individuals have specific health needs, and we want their experience here to be exceptional. When that happens, it leads to stronger business outcomes and a more inspired staff."

Institutions that are privately held or publicly traded have another stakeholder to consider, namely the shareholder or investor. People who buy stock undoubtedly want a substantial return on their investment. No one wants to invest in an institution that perpetually loses money.

Insurance, product innovation, pharmaceuticals, biotech, medical device companies, and even some hospital systems are publicly traded entities. Policymakers are elected officials who must address the needs of their constituents and get reelected. Providers must work within the system's details.

No common mission exists among the parts of our health system. Each moves according to its own momentum, rarely in sync with the others. This is what I describe as health system kinetics, the push and pull of forces that shape outcomes without coordination. We cannot dismantle the system and build anew, nor can we transform it overnight. What we can do is establish a shared focus, a common mission that guides how all players engage with one another and, most importantly, with the people they are meant to serve. We must collectively rally to the clarion call that people matter.

When your insurance is provided through the government, such as Medicare or Medicaid, do you feel confident that coverage decisions are made in your favor, rather than against you?

Does your doctor give you sufficient time to explain yourself without imposing a preconceived judgment?

Do government officials convince you that they lead by prioritizing the people who depend on the system?

Ultimately, the diverse economic structures of the five pillars are acceptable. Some are for-profit, and others are not. The issue is that they do not share a common mission.

Money should be a conduit to achieving the experience-based mission. Maintaining strength and economic viability is essential to fulfilling a human-centered mission; however, it should not be the mission itself.

Singular Planets

No matter what we might wish, the five Ps of the health system will remain. Some will argue that one P or another is not sufficiently important to be a pillar. Others will try to convince you that, for example, investors are just as important as the five Ps, when, in reality, investors are merely audiences that react to them.

The five Ps are like planets, while everything else—from investors to financial analysts—orbits around them like moons. The moons are essential, but the five Ps ultimately make up the health system.

The pillars often interact with one another. For example, if you (the patient) see your doctor (a provider) who prescribes you medicine, you will need to go to a pharmacist (another provider). Then, the pharmacist will tell you whether the medicine is covered by your health insurance, meaning you are now dealing with the payer, whose policies the government sets.

In that example, four of the five pillars are at play. Each P determines its opinion, approach, or position on your health needs, but from a financial standpoint. They are not necessarily worried about you or people like you, but about their budgets, processes, systems, and authority. No one remains focused on your well-being, thinking, "I hope that person feels better." The system, not the patient, becomes the customer of the health enterprise.

The real question is whether people will become healthier through the system's decision-making processes and spending. Too often, human-centered decisions are pushed aside. Instead, the system is consumed with balancing budgets, generating profit, securing enough patient reimbursements to cover bills, and simply keeping the doors open. The formulary people who are part of the payer might wonder, "Will we balance the budget? Will we get a better cost for these drugs?"

Industry reports often present polished lists of payer priorities. One such list prioritized "cost management" first, followed by "value-based care," shifting from fee-for-service models to ones where efficiency is rewarded over volume. Third came "population health management," emphasizing prevention and chronic disease control; yet in practice, payers rarely elevate this approach, as short-term financial pressures often dominate.

Finally, "streamlining administrative processes" rounded out the list, a goal that may reduce overhead but has little to do with improving patient experience. These curated priorities read well on paper, but they often diverge sharply from what patients and providers encounter.

What should number one have been other than "keeping people healthy"? After all, is that not the cheapest way to save money?

The government tends to focus on negotiating costs, yet far fewer efforts are made toward providing children with what they truly need for lifelong health. Simple priorities such as eating nutritious food, engaging in daily exercise, and spending more time playing instead of using screens are among the most powerful forms of prevention. For instance, when students routinely eat school meals, their diets tend to be modestly healthier.

Recent evidence suggests that after-school physical activity programs are more than just a healthy diversion;

over a two-year period, children who regularly participate in these programs exhibit measurable changes in body composition, according to a 2023 study by Alberty and colleagues. In a shorter, focused trial, a ten-week play-based intervention improved fitness, agility, and balance among twelve-year-old participants, as a 2024 study by Kurnaz and colleagues shows. Programs like nutritious school lunches and structured physical activity offer tangible proof that prevention works if only we prioritize and invest in it.

Of all five Ps, the patient has the least amount of clout.

Let us begin at the core of the system: the patient experience. Even typically benign medical procedures, such as colonoscopies, lead to worry and trepidation that we often overlook.

A doctor in the U.S. who is unaffiliated with an institution but has a private practice begins their year with a salary of zero. Their specialty does not matter. This is because we have a fee-for-service system, which means doctors can only charge patients and get reimbursed after treatment. Thus, a doctor must see many patients and use the reimbursement codes, or the “J-code,” to earn money and pay their office staff.

Working in a hospital makes earning a high salary even more challenging because hospitals are large buildings with many people and equipment. Like doctors, hospitals begin the year with a revenue line of zero. They require many people to come through their doors and provide services.

This explains why payers can assume doctors are performing medically unnecessary procedures to generate revenue. Thus, the payers keep a keen eye out for what is necessary. They have a preauthorization system that requires you to obtain their approval before undergoing an X-ray, MRI, or blood test. Similarly, doctors need to send prescription orders to insurance companies for authorization.

Meanwhile, you, the patient, have to wonder if the insurance company will provide authorization. You live within that question. You most likely feel anxious because your doctor, whom you trust, has explained why this or that medical treatment is necessary. What if the doctor does not receive permission?

All of these considerations center on the cost of health innovation, which is regulated by policymakers—in other words, the government. No matter who you are, the government agencies that administer beneficiary services, such as Medicare and Medicaid, make those policy determinations and set the course of action.

The pillars are not in harmony. It is almost as if they are playing a game of pickup basketball. Everyone is playing, but on different teams.

I have a colonoscopy every five years, a standard test that is always authorized. Afterward, I received a bill that you would think my insurance company covers as a given. However, at that time, the anesthesiologist's work was not covered, as my insurance company did not consider them a provider. In the meantime, I was left to argue with both the GI practice and the insurance company.

It's ridiculous! Why is my gastroenterologist a provider, but not my anesthesiologist, participating in the same procedure? I did not select my anesthesiologist. My gastroenterologist knows my insurance company because they reimburse him. Somehow, my anesthesiologist is separate. Thus, the gastroenterology center sends me a bill for the cost of my anesthesiologist. I have no choice in this situation.

My wife and I argued back in response, saying, “Hey, this is not our problem. You know our insurance company. You knew how you would be reimbursed. Choose an anesthesiologist who is covered by my insurance. It’s not me who chooses them, but you.”

Who would choose to have a colonoscopy without anesthesia? No one! Even if you had the option, you are unlikely to agree to be strapped down to a gurney during the procedure. Nothing about a colonoscopy without anesthesia is customer-friendly or supportive of the gastroenterology practice.

Gastroenterologists do not receive substantial reimbursement for colonoscopies. They must perform several procedures before earning a profit, as they first have to cover the costs of equipment, sterilization, and staff. Recent policy changes have finally addressed one of the most frustrating gaps: patients being billed separately for an out-of-network anesthesiologist during an otherwise routine, in-network colonoscopy. That bureaucratic tangle has largely been corrected. Perhaps someone finally asked, “What if this happened to me?” and decided it was time to fix it.

The more we squeeze the cost of the health system, the more doctors say, “I don’t want to be a doctor anymore.

It's too much of a hassle." Then, more private practice doctors sell their practices to institutions that will manage the administration or payer on their behalf.

This way, the health system and its experience become an unpleasant commodity. Like any nagging problem, it becomes the can that is kicked down the road toward the patient, who is powerless to fix the problem.

Can We Focus on Why the System Exists?

My critique of the health system stems from my love for people who work tirelessly to heal and help others. I also don't want to suggest that radical change is required, given the disruption that would cause. I want to highlight the great benefits that could be realized if every piece of the system shared a common code centered on the patient experience.

Dr. Alison Grann at St. Barnabas in Livingston, New Jersey, fundamentally understands that her staff sets the tone and culture of patient and consumer care. People feel welcomed because their needs are built into the system's structure and culture. She and her staff know people rarely want to visit a hospital or see a doctor, even though they need to. Their experience should be positive and comfortable, which would require not arguing with an insurance company. You immediately feel they respect your time. Even the possibility of a wait is taken seriously, accompanied by a proactive apology.

Dr. Grann and her staff aim to treat each patient like a 1K passenger on an airline. I'm a 1K flyer on United Airlines. If I ask a question, mention a seat or a meal, or talk about a flight, no one says, "We will not authorize that." Instead, they respond, "Thank you for being a 1K flyer." They show respect to the customer.

Often, patients are treated as bothersome rather than as people the system exists to serve. Too often, avoidance stems not from the complexity of their illness but from the anxiety and fear that shape their behavior. Many of these patients live with what can only be described as "medical PTSD," deep weariness and dread born of repeated, difficult encounters with the system.

Instead of meeting this anxiety with empathy, the anxious, chronically ill, and frequent ER visitors are too often labeled as "problems." Rarely does a provider or payer pause to say, "I see you've been in the hospital a lot lately. That must be terrifying. What can I do to support you? I'll tell you what I can do, but first, I want to understand what you would like to see happen."

If that patient replies, "I need to see a consulting gastroenterologist," a provider could say, "I will put in a request right now. It may take some time for them to arrive based on patient priorities, but I will put in the request and come back to confirm to you I've sent it."

Patients rarely feel that someone is advocating for them. Instead, they feel pushed aside. At best, a more typical response to that patient request might be, "You know, we're swamped. You can see our ER is very busy. We'll get to you as quickly as we can."

Factors contributing to a person's health, such as environmental or social factors, are part of what I refer to as "Health System Kinetics." The concept of kinetics is the relationship between things. It is pattern recognition. Imagine looking at a Lego piece and trying to determine where it fits.

In America, the system seems to dismiss this concept altogether. Health system kinetics describes the dynamic forces at play within the health ecosystem—the constant push and pull among the five Ps: patients, payers, policymakers, product innovators, and providers. These pillars are always in motion, shaping and influencing one another. When aligned, they create momentum toward better outcomes. When misaligned, they generate friction, inefficiency, and frustration.

Like assembling a complex Lego set, each piece has its place. The structure weakens if one is missing or forced into the wrong spot. The same is true of our health system. Patients, payers, providers, policymakers, and innovators each have their role, but without connection and alignment, the whole system wobbles.

Health system kinetics challenges us to recognize these interdependencies and intentionally direct them toward a common mission. When money and mission are seen as complementary rather than contradictory, progress accelerates. Caregivers are supported, innovation is sustained, and ultimately, people receive better health because they matter.

Fragmentation is partly caused by ignoring the impact of social factors on health. We must develop a new way of thinking that acknowledges health kinetics surrounding human health. That could include studying not only planetary health but also how the health of other regions could influence us. It would enable us to contemplate the influence of economic well-being on health more seriously.

Currently, we consider everything to be a one-off experience. We have a "whack-a-mole" system. When a problem arises, we merely whitewash it over. When another similar problem crops up, we whack that one, too, and so on. Not enough people say, "We didn't have all these problems before. Maybe we can avoid, preempt, and prevent some of them by focusing on people's experience."

In my article about the assassination of Brian Thompson, I argue that the health industry should engage in the discussion about how to better serve consumers. More than that, in response to people applauding a murderer and plastering billboards with "Who's next?", it clearly needs to change.

This killing represents pent-up public ire. Public outcry is typically the next step toward enacting legislation that addresses a pressing problem. Unless the industry begins to engage and demonstrates that it hears the bubbling outrage, the resentment and anger will grow.

Since the advent of managed care, these issues have consistently persisted. The difference is that they have recently been placed under a magnifying glass. It is unbelievable that our reaction to an assassination is, "Hmm, should we do something about this?" instead of, "Wait a minute. What took us so long? Why don't we act proactively?"

The reasons for this lack of proactive action are economics and the comfort of the status quo. Many people say, "Let's stick to how we do things as long as we can because it will deliver profits." We need a vision to move past the status quo.

I often return to a quote by George W. Merck, who led the company that bears his family's name through the mid-20th century. Speaking as a keynote at the Medical College of Virginia in 1950, he said, "We try never to forget that medicine is for the people." To this day, Merck executives, including legendary leaders such as Roy Vagelos, MD, and Ken Frazier, have upheld this vision.

Merck's era of greatest respect and profitability was when its mission centered on the idea that addressing people's needs would lead to financial success. During that time, the company donated billions of dollars' worth of medicine to treat onchocerciasis, also known as river blindness, worldwide. That disease has nearly disappeared thanks to Merck's generosity and its partnership with the Carter Center, ensuring that medical supplies reached the people in need.

Imagine if every pharmaceutical company followed Jonas Salk's example and offered the patent for the polio vaccine to the public. Today, no company would donate its medicine outright because it would lose money. However, a company can still earn profit while addressing the needs of a population if it creates partnerships that channel medicine in a way that ensures cost recovery.

Imagine if the industry and payers began to see mission and money as intertwined. They might say, "These people are severely ill and cost us a lot of money. However, if we proactively engage with them and assign them a caseworker, they will improve."

When social workers step in early and proactively engage families with high needs, the impact is striking; hospital admissions have been shown to decline by up to 50 percent and emergency-room visits decrease significantly, according to a 2022 Commonwealth Fund analysis. Savings exceed $1,300 per patient each year; far more than the $60,000 average annual earnings of a social worker. The result is fewer crises, lower costs, and families who feel supported rather than abandoned.

Sometimes, the best intervention for a child with asthma isn't another ER visit, but an air conditioner. We need to change our mindset so that we automatically ask, "What would happen to my family? My child? What would I want?" This kind of questioning can lead to a deeper understanding of health kinetics. It can also allow us to find the capacity for empathetic decision-making within ourselves.

The system must ask itself, "What can we do to sustain and save lives?" instead of, "How do we manage our government budget, our hospital's budget, the payer's profitability, and the oncology department's budget?"

We remain too focused on the system's structural aspects instead of its mission. That's not to say we should ignore structure; rather, we should view it through the lens of purpose.

A successful business requires human leadership. I created a business not by myself, but in harmony with others. I am the leader, but I am also a catalyst. I brought in people who believed in my vision and were willing to partner with me to bring it to life.

The FINN Global Health Practice, which I am privileged to lead, is part of FINN Partners, founded by Peter Finn. His vision is to build an agency with a heart and a conscience—one that makes a difference. A decade ago, the Practice was little more than a mandate and a handful of committed colleagues. Today, it has evolved into a multi-million-dollar business unit.

This progress does not belong to me; it belongs to the clients and the people who chose this culture and built it together. I am grateful to help convene that talent and to keep us aligned to the mission. Culture attracts a certain kind of person, and when culture leads, performance follows. Healthcare has a culture, too. When economics eclipse it, we lose what makes the work meaningful.

In the 14th century, priests began to found Christian hospices. What medicine did the clergy have at that time? They didn't say, "This person has a bacterial infection—should we authorize an antibiotic?" They had no antibiotics or other medicines. Caring was the only form of healing they could offer. They could provide soup, a cold compress, a bed, and their own presence—priests or other healers willing to put themselves at risk.

Why? Because they wanted to help people. At the core of humanity is the desire of healers to help those who seek healing.

Culturally, we must return to that core desire. Everyone working within the health system needs to be inspired by the administrators at the payer level, nurses in the trenches, those in laboratories inventing new medicines, physicians at the bedside, patient advocates, and policymakers. At the core, we must say, "I am here. My mission is to help you get better. If you can't get better, my mission is to help you on your journey to the end with care."

In 2017, the future of the Affordable Care Act, also known as Obamacare, was being debated in the Senate. The president sought to repeal it. Surprisingly, a leading Republican, Senator John McCain, voted against overturning Obamacare. Why? He had brain cancer. He knew he was dying. He had compassion and recognized that minimal or no health coverage is tantamount to a rapid death sentence.

You could interpret his vote as saying, "Look at me. I have access to care because I'm a United States Senator. I have government health insurance, which is among the best in the nation. Why would I strip away health insurance from the people who have the least?"

Being patient-centered begins with empathy. While economic performance is a valid system metric, we also need one that reflects the patient's lived experience. Healthcare should measure success not only by finances but also by whether patients feel heard, respected, and supported. The goal must be to move beyond dwelling on problems and instead focus on solutions—creating a system where empathy and care are intertwined.

We also can't bring the system to a screeching halt and stop treating people until we figure out the best path forward. We can't say, "No one goes to the hospital for the next three months. The dying will die. The sick will get sicker."

We cannot rebuild an airplane mid-flight. What we can do is slowly train and reorient the culture around health kinetics and people. We need to inspire healers to want to heal those who seek healing.

Creating a culture of celebration that centers on healing, appreciation, and empathy requires a commitment to education. In medical schools, future doctors must be taught that caring is part of the healthcare package. Hospital systems must determine the cause of provider burnout. Patients must be heard. Nurses' grueling routines must be reconsidered.

We must examine sickness hotspots in the U.S., such as Camden, New Jersey, which already bears an alarmingly high disease burden. Camden County's 2020 premature death rate was 567.9 per 100,000, significantly higher than many other counties nationally. Much of this excess mortality is driven by the forces of poverty, chronic illness, unstable housing, and limited access to preventive care. Clearly, what we are doing now is insufficient.

We need to move past the approach of treating the patient as they are and adopt the mindset of determining why the patient is sick in the first place.

Families relying on food assistance often face limited access to healthy options, even as rates of diabetes rise. Our programs should not disproportionately subsidize processed foods that are high in sugar and fat, regardless of how cheap and filling they may be. In some inner-city communities, fresh produce is so rare that people may never encounter foods like nectarines.

This is not about individual choice, but about what the system makes affordable and available. When healthy food is out of reach financially or geographically, it is no surprise that chronic illness flourishes. That is health system kinetics in action.

We opt to deal with sickness rather than prevent it. We have a sick care system instead of a health system. Transforming our sick care system into a health system requires financing and a shared and prioritized mission for each of the system's pieces.

I believe in the power of a thoughtfully regulated market because free enterprise, when guided by responsibility, can drive remarkable progress. At the same time, people come first. I do not wish to dismantle the system or spend more. However, we need to ask whether the resources we already invest are aimed at the real causes of our health challenges. We must take a hard look at how and when we utilize our money, talent, and innovation, ensuring they serve the mission of improving lives.

I also believe that government-sponsored systems can be effective. Regardless, I want to prioritize people as the center of the system because people are the reason the system exists in the first place.

We must also appreciate and celebrate particularly empathetic and engaged individuals, such as Albert

Schweitzer, the renowned humanitarian physician who worked in Africa. Films and books have been written about him. We celebrate Jonas Salk, Paul Janssen, Roy Vagelos, and George W. Merck because they inspire us with their vision and ability to build innovative cultures. Yet, we also value any given CEO because our shareholder dividend is strong.

Why can't we create CEOs who deliver strong shareholder returns while also inspiring greater collective health results? We know it is possible; leaders who walk confidently on the path of purpose and profit already exist. The real question is, why don't we celebrate them as the gold standard to which others should aspire?

Sadly, we have become so accustomed to the system's breakdown that we no longer expect anything better. That must change.

Chapter 3

THE TOLL OF EXHAUSTION ON PATIENTS AND CARE PROVIDERS

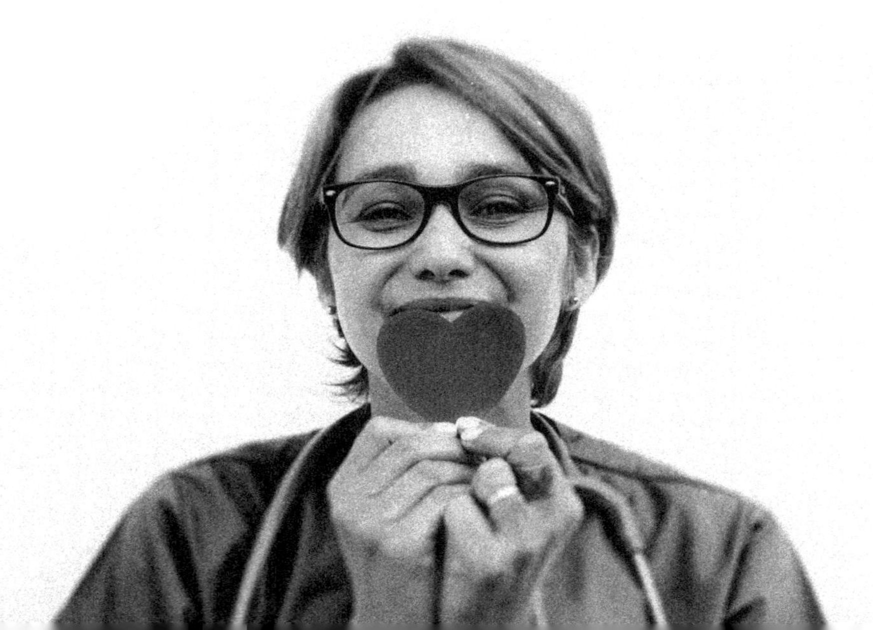

MANY health professionals have hung up their white coats and stethoscopes in the wake of the COVID-19 pandemic. Obstetricians, gynecologists, OB-GYNs, primary care physicians, internists, hospitalists, and nurses continue to leave the field.

These dramatic career decisions are not anomalies. They are part of a broader pattern in which health professionals, once drawn to the calling of healing, are pushed away by the bureaucratic burden.

I have spoken to several doctors who have left medicine to pursue careers in fields far removed from their medical training. I know one OB-GYN who went into real estate. I know two orthopedic surgeons who left the surgery suite and are happily evaluating workers' compensation claims. Their passion for medicine was extinguished not by the pressure of patient demands but by the reams of paperwork required by a demanding reimbursement system.

The pressure to manage a medical practice has escalated to such an extent that a urologist I have known for decades, who loved caring for his patients, closed his practice because he could no longer tolerate the hoops of third-party insurance's prior authorization requirements. He could no longer deal with the headaches required to work with payers. He said negotiating with “actuaries” added hours to each day and delayed care.

For many, going through medical school is inspired by the motivation to do something meaningful and make a difference. Something draws them to become healers. Over the years, many have shared with me their experiences of loss, including the loss of a parent, sibling, or teacher, which compelled them to answer the call to be healers. Nurses, doctors, and emergency medical technicians enjoy their clinical work. However, through the years, they have found it painfully difficult to maintain that inspirational spark in their day-to-day work lives.

Operating within the health ecosystem has become a labyrinth. The paperwork, liability, and administrative shepherding needed in modern medicine have become an albatross. Simply put, healers are burning out.

As noted in other chapters, not-for-profit health systems such as Ascension, CommonSpirit Health, Cooper University Health Care, Kaiser Permanente, and Mass General Brigham consistently report strong patient outcomes and higher staff morale. Though they represent only a fraction of hospitals nationwide, their scores for patient experience and employee satisfaction stand out.

One reason behind these results is how these systems manage administrative demands. They often place the burden of compliance and reporting on dedicated administrative teams, people who find meaning in "keeping the ship afloat." This frees physicians, nurses, and other health professionals to focus on where they belong: with patients, not with spreadsheets.

The irony is hard to miss. At the very moment when medical science is delivering breathtaking breakthroughs in cancer care, obesity treatment, and other fields, non-medical requirements are draining clinicians' enthusiasm and driving many from practice. It raises a question that Jim Collins asked in his 2001 bestseller Good to Great: Do we have the right people on the bus, and are they in the right seats?

Too often, physicians, nurses, and allied health professionals are assigned to roles that are buried under paperwork instead of ones where their skills can directly benefit patients. The same misalignment is true across the ecosystem: innovators focus on regulatory checklists, payers on cost containment, and policymakers on partisan wins. The bus is full of brilliant people, but if we don't seat them to serve the patient as the destination, we risk driving in circles.

Working with electronic medical records is arduous and daunting. By law, case reports must be filled out after or during every patient visit. What was once a calling to heal has become, in many respects, a part-time job in paperwork. Too often, doctors end their day only to begin another shift, typing notes late into the night or dictating notes for transcription that may come back incomplete or inaccurate.

Hospitals depend on highly educated, well-paid professionals to maintain quality standards. Healthcare is, at its heart, a people-driven business operating on thin margins. We would expect service—how well patients feel cared for to be the differentiator. Instead, the perception is that the system seems to value completed paperwork more than it values the patient experience.

Technology holds the promise of relief, yet it often creates new burdens. Every advancement raises the same essential question: Does this tool bring doctor and patient closer together, or does it push them further apart? Large language models are beginning to move us toward a better place, translating data into actionable insights that meet human needs. But for too long, health record systems such as Epic and other EHRs failed to ease the real work of medicine: spending time with patients and thinking deeply about their cases.

The problem is not only the technology but also the people and processes wrapped around it. Electronic health records were designed to promote collaboration. Yet, even today, two doctors practicing less than a mile apart, or even in the same building, struggle to share information on the same patient. The burden of connection falls on patients themselves, who shuttle from office to office, serving as their own couriers to keep the care team informed.

We are closing that gap because generative AI can be programmed to scrape information from large databases, servers, or the general internet. This can enable more efficient interactions between medical professionals and technology, but only if we remain vigilant for AI-related hallucinations, which require human cognition and patient engagement.

While the process is improving, it remains ineffective to have doctors performing data entry tasks instead of attending to patients. Doctors want to be healers. Between the hospital systems and the payer system, the challenge of data entry remains. Current administrative strategies have created unnecessary obstacles, which we are now starting to address to make medicine more focused on patients.

We need to spend our time and attention on patients. Instead, we have made administrative work so demanding that it rivals the healing process itself. During a visit, our doctors are often looking at their laptop screens, rather than looking at us. That isn't their choice. It's what they must do to weather the system.

These challenges are not abstract; they touch daily lives. In my own family, we often see how payer systems erode the compassionate spirit of providers because it just wears people out. This is not just anecdotal. As recently as May 2025, the American Medical Association reported that more than 40 percent of U.S. healthcare professionals experience symptoms of burnout, and studies have linked burnout to a twofold increase in medical errors and higher turnover rates. The impacts are both personal and professional.

Even the politest person will find their patience stretched to the limit in frustration when speaking with their insurance carrier. We all wonder if these companies invest in training their staff on the other side of our calls in human dynamics. Are the people who administer health insurance coached in the same way we would train someone working in a consumer retail store about customer experience? Are payer staff being trained to be attuned to the customer's experience?

We could universally say there isn't enough training or support to provide a health insurance representative with the background and skills needed to hold a meaningful conversation that leads to a positive experience. When we're on the phone with a payer's representative, we need someone who is listening, engaging, and caring. As consumers, we need to feel that our concerns are taken seriously. We need to feel valued, and the person representing the insurance company should be inspired to do good work as an ambassador.

Are we training people to ensure their connection with the patient is meaningful, beneficial, and positive? Patient experience data say we are not. One Forbes article suggests that 60 percent of Americans report having had a negative healthcare experience in recent years.

When dealing with the system as a patient, it's human to feel anxiety before we walk in. We find an automatic built-in level of anxiety. That is a human dynamic. We're not going to the doctor because it's a terrific experience or because we're feeling in tip-top shape and want to report how good we feel to the doctor.

Beyond physical health, the primary reason we visit the doctor is that something is not right in our lives. The doctor enters the conversation knowing we have concerns. They must take sufficient time and bandwidth to engage us in addressing our situation and finding an effective path forward.

When my doctor recently ordered lab tests, the samples were sent to a diagnostic lab my insurance plan doesn't cover. The result: an $800 bill. Had the office used my payer's preferred lab, I would have owed nothing, as my copay requirements were already met. Now, we faced the uphill battle to get this surprise bill covered.

How did this leave me feeling as a patient and customer? Frustrated, invisible, and stuck. My doctor knows my insurance carrier. Someone in the office should have caught this, but didn't. Given the substantial amount of money spent on software, a basic program should have flagged it automatically. Instead, I'm left asking: Who is responsible for the $800—the doctor, the payer, or me?

Well, no need to leave you hanging. I'm responsible for the bill.

This is the everyday reality for patients. Instead of confidence, interactions with the health system often leave people feeling powerless. The system shrugs while patients carry the burden. That's the deeper problem: in these moments, it becomes painfully clear that the patient is not the system's customer. The customer is the system itself. Until that changes, stories like this will continue to repeat and trust will continue to erode.

The health system customer is now the steward of the process. We're paying for fine dining and having to go into the kitchen, cook the meal, and serve ourselves. I'm now responsible for consolidating my health records across various provider platforms and ensuring that my budget remains in the black, as the health industry has essentially outsourced customer service to its own customers and charged them for the privilege.

A few decades back, a sales pitch indicated that computerizing our health records would make addressing our personal health journey easier. We have technology, but the promise of technology making our lives better has been elusive. Little modern medical technology exists to enhance the patient experience.

Patients today have been reduced to numbers on spreadsheets. Health is no longer measured in people's lives but in dollars. My well-being feels secondary to the administrative management of my case. Every month, I hand over a significant portion of my income to my insurance company. In return, I'm granted the "privilege" of fighting to access what I've already paid for. They are not partners in my health; they are another closed door I'm forced to pry open. Customer service hasn't simply been outsourced; it's been dumped on the customer. As a result, our expectations of fairness have sunk to almost nothing.

Doctors feel this same strain. When they sit with me, they're not only thinking about my health; they're also thinking about how to document every detail to ensure reimbursement. At this pace, a medical visit becomes less about healing and more about checking boxes in a fee-for-service world. The human connection, the core of medicine, has slipped into the background, replaced by a relentless pursuit of profit.

When I speak about great physicians, I mean those who rise above the system. These are the professionals who never lose sight of medicine's true north: people first, paperwork second. They understand the system but refuse to let it dictate their compassion. These are the doctors who keep the patient—not the process—at the center of care.

Ideally, if you have access, seek out that kind of health professional: someone who remains aligned with true north and who understands that medicine is, above all else, about people. Hospitals and health systems must follow that same compass. From a customer experience perspective, staff should be trained not only in clinical skill but also in the art of prioritizing the human encounter—because empathy and trust lead to better outcomes.

The evidence is clear. Patients who feel connected to their care experience less anxiety, engage more actively, and adhere more consistently to treatment plans. A meta-analysis of 47 studies found that patients who trust their health professionals demonstrate significantly better health behaviors, higher quality of life, and greater satisfaction with care, real-life evidence underscored by neuroscience researcher Johanna Birkhäuer and her colleagues in 2017 in their study "Trust in the Health Care Professional and Health Outcomes."

Another review linked trust to improved mental health outcomes, including lower rates of depression and anxiety among people with chronic disease.

Trust is not a soft metric. It is the foundation of healing. So why is it so rare in our health system? Because the system increasingly treats itself, rather than the patient, as the customer. When the focus drifts from people, empathy drifts with it.

Health system kinetics today rarely influence the thinking or operations of the players in the field. The system's goal should be to meet medical needs while managing the supply chain for sustainability and effectiveness. However, the essential question remains: are we prioritizing the experience of the patient and the health professional—or the comfort of the administrative overseer, as in Yes, Minister?

We must also ask whether the technology being developed today truly enhances the experiences of those on the frontlines of care—physicians, nurses, pharmacists, and patients alike. Insurance companies, too, must examine how they communicate with beneficiaries: are their letters and emails written in language that people can easily understand, or do they create yet another barrier to trust?

Currently, we are doing very little of this. It is time for some basic, prescriptive changes.

Insurance companies should consider appointing chief engagement officers supported by teams dedicated to evaluating whether customer service genuinely champions the customer. Does the experience make people feel safe, valued, confident, and heard? Do patients believe they can successfully navigate the reimbursement process? These are not abstract ideals; they are the building blocks of trust.

Insurance companies are not usually invested in customer experience because their customer isn't the patient, but the buyer of the insurance, most often the patient's employer.

Hospitals should take a similar approach. When someone faces a severe illness, a dedicated staff member should be assigned to help that patient and their family manage the journey. If the patient is indeed the customer, then the patient experience must become the primary metric of success.

A simple analogy illustrates why this matters. In a major retail clothing store, customer experience is paramount. Imagine someone asking, "Excuse me, can you tell me where the men's department is?" There are two possible responses. One is, "Let me show you." The other is, "There's a sign near the elevator."

This distinction matters.

At NYU Langone, I once asked for directions to a particular department. A doctor replied, "It's hard to find. Let me show you." He walked me halfway there and said, "Now you're on the right path—it's just down that hallway." That brief moment of kindness made a lasting impression.

Contrast that with the alternative: if an employee pointed to a sign and told you to follow it, would you want to shop there again? Probably not. However, if

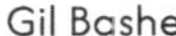

they took the time to guide you, you'd remember that store whenever you needed something in the future. The same principle applies to healthcare. A few moments of empathy can transform a patient's experience.

The more patient-friendly we make the system, the better customers feel about what is already a frightening experience. Conversely, when care feels purely transactional, patients feel less valued and start looking for alternatives if they have them. This erosion of spirit contributes directly to the broader crisis we now recognize as burnout.

Burnout

In 2022, nearly half of health workers, 46 percent, reported experiencing burnout often or very often, according to the Centers for Disease Control and Prevention. The causes are no mystery: long hours, heavy patient loads, emotional strain, endless paperwork, and a system that leaves little time for true healing.

When people are burned out, they do not perform at their best. Some argue that those who tire should never have chosen a career in medicine. However, when nearly half of physicians and nurses report exhaustion, the issue is not a personal weakness; it is a systemic failure. Burnout at this scale is not a lack of resilience; it is the collapse of structure.

Payers must recognize that providers are not cost centers to be managed; they are the foundation of a sound health system. A rested and supported physician delivers better outcomes at a lower cost for both patients and payers. Health system kinetics should be centered on people. When the system serves only itself, it ultimately destroys itself.

Patients feel this collapse as much as providers do. Many reach a breaking point and say, “I can’t deal with this anymore.” One man, Forrest VanPatten, was just 50 years old when he died. Among many other heartbreaking narratives, he conveys that he spent the last hours of his life arguing with his insurance company for cancer treatment. This is what happens when bureaucracy replaces empathy. People stop fighting—not because of their illness, but because the system makes hope seem impossible.

Cancer treatment is grueling. There is nothing unreasonable about a 97-year-old saying, “I’ve lived a long life; I’m ready to let go.” It is understandable for someone with late-stage terminal cancer to choose palliative care. However, when younger patients or those with treatable diseases give up because they feel abandoned by an uncaring, faceless system, that is not medicine; it is betrayal.

Patients with advanced cancer should receive the care they need within a supportive system. Their families should not have to navigate mountains of paperwork, and physicians should have the time and motivation to deliver high-quality care. When people feel that their lives lack quality, it is understandable that the end of life starts to look like relief.

On a recent episode of the podcast Straight Outta Health IT with Christopher Kunney, I described palliative care as a clinical option that should be introduced at the right time. It is a decision rooted in clarity—recognizing when the human experience is nearing its close and when the next stage may bring pain and suffering. In those moments, patients and families deserve to know they can choose comfort, dignity, and compassionate support until life's final day.

Yet too often, this option is overlooked due to system fragmentation. Doctors worry that raising the subject of palliative care will make them appear less encouraging or hopeful, so the conversation happens late in the treatment cycle. That silence robs patients of choice.

Palliative care should never be an afterthought. It belongs within the decision-making process as a vital expression of empathy and humanity. When patients turn to palliative care only because they can no longer endure unmanaged pain, that is not good medicine; it is evidence that the system has failed. The responsibility to relieve suffering should not fall solely on the patient's endurance or the physician's shoulders.

The American Medical Association notes that physicians who feel more positive about their profession also feel more engaged in their work and are less vulnerable to burnout. This is more than a statistic; it is a signal. When the system fails to prioritize empathy, it fails both patients and doctors. Supporting physicians in balancing hope with honesty—and giving them the time and resources to address suffering—not only preserves patient dignity but also protects doctors from the corrosive effects of burnout.

The question is simple but urgent: how do we build a system that keeps physicians on track to do their best work? Too often, technology has been part of the problem. Clunky electronic health records and documentation requirements add hours of administrative work, contributing to widespread burnout among clinicians. Poorly designed health IT is repeatedly cited as a leading driver of exhaustion and disengagement.

Burnout is not only emotional fatigue, it is also the collision of compassion and complexity. Physicians enter medicine to heal, not to code and click. Yet many spend more hours documenting care than delivering it, trapped in a cycle of forms, denials, and digital noise that erodes both purpose and joy.

Consider the GLP-1 wave of medications. These treatments hold extraordinary promise in reducing cardiovascular risk and helping patients with obesity and diabetes avoid cascading comorbidities. According to a nationwide American Medical Association 2023 physician survey, practices complete an average of 39 prior-authorization requests per physician per week, and physicians and their staff spend roughly 13 hours weekly completing these requests.

Navigating paperwork tied to GLP-1 prescribing places additional administrative strain that nearly nine in ten health professionals link to burnout. When doctors are bogged down in paperwork instead of providing front-line care, they lose time, energy, emotional reserves, and revenue. When that happens, patients who could

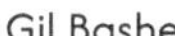

benefit most are left waiting. If we hope to bend the cost curve and restore trust in care, physicians must be positioned as part of the solution, not an afterthought.

This is not a story about a single drug. It is a symptom of a larger condition. When progress meets bureaucracy, innovation becomes another source of exhaustion rather than empowerment. If we want to heal burnout, we must design systems that reward both compassion and efficiency, rather than pitting them against each other. Supporting physicians is not kindness; it is essential infrastructure for better care.

Technology can also be part of the solution. Take exam smart rooms, for example. With ambient digital tools that "listen" to the patient–physician interaction, a visit can be automatically recorded, summarized, and a transcript provided to both the physician and patient before they leave. This provides an opportunity to review next steps.

Early pilots at Mass General Brigham demonstrated a 21 percent decrease in burnout prevalence in just under three months, while Emory's program showed a 30 percent increase in documentation-related well-being within 60 days. These innovations don't just save time; they restore focus to where it belongs—human connection.

Yet, technology alone will not solve burnout. It must be designed and implemented with purpose. It must be perfected to ensure accuracy. That requires real investment of time, energy, and intention to ensure that every tool reduces burdens on health professionals rather than adds to their already constrained workday.

Recently, during a routine visit, my mother-in-law mentioned that her late husband had lived with multiple myeloma. The in-room transcription system misheard it, and when my wife checked her mother's electronic record that evening, that passing comment had become her diagnosis. It was a sharp reminder that while technology can streamline care, errors can move just as quickly and once they enter the record, they can be hard to unwind.

Patients as Widgets

To understand how far medicine has drifted from its original purpose, consider the roots of hospice care. In the Middle Ages, churches established hospices as sanctuaries where the ill and dying could spend their final days with dignity and respect. Priests, monks, and nuns offered presence, comfort, and compassion—medicine in its purest form. Healing then was less about science and more about humanity.

That legacy stands in stark contrast to parts of today's system, where patients are too often processed like "widgets." The message is implicit: I'm the doctor, you're the patient. I hold the authority; you are the broken inferior. I'm not here to see you as a person, but to move you through insurance rules and liability checklists.

This shift from compassion to transaction is not inevitable; it's a cultural choice. Remembering hospice's origins reminds us that care begins not with forms or formulas but with empathy, dignity, and the recognition that every patient is more than a chart or a claim.

At its core, providing healthcare is both a service and a privilege. However, when doctors lose their compass and begin to believe it's about them, where does the patient fit in? If a patient takes the initiative in their care experience, the doctor may feel slighted because the standard protocol wasn't followed.

I once encountered a situation where a six-lead ECG test yielded an unexpected and concerning result, although it ultimately proved benign. I scheduled an echocardiogram at a convenient time that wouldn't conflict with an upcoming trip. When I later visited my primary care physician to request a prescription for the echo, she was not pleased that I had taken the initiative. She felt she was being ordered to act rather than being consulted.

Meanwhile, I had already spoken with my cardiologist, Dr. Larry Phillips, who immediately said, "Absolutely, you need an echo. Where are you having it done? I'll call in a prescription."

Two doctors, two different reactions, two different ways of responding to my needs. Is that medicine? No—that's personality and ego at play. One empowers the patient; the other seeks to be a gatekeeper.

Medicine is not only a system of computers and data. It's a people-to-people system. It's about personalities and mindset. The job of the health system and health professionals is to inspire healthy behaviors that lead to healthier lives.

Preventive care has broken down because the doctor has limited minutes available per patient and must see a given number of cases daily. There is no time to speak to you about your diet or why you're ten pounds overweight, even though it affects your A1C, blood glucose, blood pressure, and cholesterol.

A doctor could solve several more clinical problems if they had a little more time to work with patients.

Of course, as we've seen, there is also the matter of dealing with the insurance company. If someone is overweight and has a high BMI, it would be helpful if doctors had the authority to prescribe a GLP-1 if indicated and reimburse a dietitian. However, this does not happen. They are not focused on managing your health; they're focused on managing your case.

How many people who have low PSA numbers present with prostate cancer symptoms that are missed until the cancer advances, because the physician hasn't been given time to think through the implications for that patient? If they previously presented with a 0.5 PSA one year and now it's at 1.5 a year later, that is still clinically low, but it represents a threefold jump. The doctor doesn't necessarily have the time to think through these cases.

This unyielding pressure from the system affects the doctor's judgment. How can we ensure that doctors have enough time to consider the person they treat? The same pressures extend beyond the exam room into the boardroom, where administrators and executives grapple with financial mysteries divorced from patient concerns.

Gil Bashe

Harried and Busy

Several years ago, I had the privilege of moderating conversations with industry executives, hospital leaders, and the CEOs of major companies and hospital systems. We could not discuss pricing, as it is against the law; however, we could discuss business models.

As these conversations progressed, it became clear that the different segments of our healthcare system do not have a clear view into each other's business models.

Hospital systems and physicians' practices operate on razor-thin margins. Yet, we still lack a comprehensive understanding of the true economics of the health delivery supply chain—the time, cost, and expertise that make care possible.

Consider something as simple as a branded T-shirt. The company is aware of every step in the chain, from where the cotton is grown to the cost of dye, production, packaging, and shipping. Buyers know the wholesale cost, and retailers can set an exact markup. Nothing is hidden.

Health delivery could not be more different. Yes, there are set prices for equipment and supplies, but these are layered with additional costs, including salaries, administrative overhead, sanitation, security, and technology expenses. Supplies come from around the world, each with different markups. Insurers reimburse at varying rates. Doctors and hospitals charge differently for the same procedure, depending on market dynamics or the provider's skill level. Payers enter volume deals with specific institutions. The result is a maze of costs with no clear map and almost no transparency.

If we were to open a brand-new hospital today, we could not confidently predict what its services would cost, what revenue streams it could rely on, or what reimbursements it would receive. Unlike the T-shirt, the math of medicine is a complex and mysterious field. Patients and providers live with the consequences of that opacity.

This is where the analogy to Apollo 13 comes full circle. NASA solved its crisis because every expert in Mission Control understood the problem, spoke the same technical language, and worked toward the same goal. Our health system rarely enjoys that kind of clarity. Payers, providers, innovators, and policymakers all hold pieces of the puzzle but seldom share them. The result is a fragmented system where financial blind spots undermine patient care.

If we are serious about improving health delivery, reducing costs, and enhancing care, we must stop treating everything as a black box. For some sectors of the health industry, silence is profit. We need open communication across the entire supply chain, linking hospitals, payers, product innovators, and regulators in transparent dialogue. Only then can we align resources to purpose, and profit to people. Without that collaboration, the system will continue to run on mystery instead of mission.

These problems are amplified by region. A hospital in an affluent area where people have very good insurance will likely be well reimbursed. A hospital system in rural America, or one serving an impoverished region with

Medicaid as its primary health safety net, will receive minimal reimbursement.

In Mississippi, where nearly one in four residents is enrolled in Medicaid, hospitals in low-income areas can struggle financially. Some rural hospitals now face Medicaid reimbursement gaps so severe that they threaten the institutions' very survival. A recent analysis by Families USA in 2025 indicates that independent rural hospitals could lose more than half of their net income, with an average decline of 56 percent, due to Medicaid cuts.

If Medicaid reimbursement is cut, these hospitals could close. Some people live four hours or more away from a hospital. If they experience a life-threatening medical event, and a helicopter is not available nearby, they may not survive.

This mystery around distribution and cost is part of the supply chain of care. It differs from state to state, institution to institution, and payer to payer.

Few people understand how or why medicines are priced. No system shows the costs incurred for specific periods, the expense of trials, the length of a patent, or the profit margin on a particular drug. In light of that reality, how would investors be expected to determine the best medicines to develop?

For doctors, every day brings new challenges to resolve, but for patients, each encounter is often the most important moment in their care journey. A doctor thinks, "As your physician, I already know the pathway to diagnose you, but I have to negotiate with the insurance company to get them to approve my diagnostic path way. After diagnosis, I'll then need to get an agreement to reimburse me for treating you and to sustain you if there is long-term chronic care treatment."

Think about the responsibility on a doctor's shoulders. When they were young adults aspiring to become doctors, it was all about treating patients. Now, they must also be masters of the health supply chain and cost management.

This is among the reasons why many doctors or group practices sell themselves to hospital systems. They were making money before, but it is far more efficient for the hospital to manage the administration and reimbursement process. The small practice welcomes the opportunity to shed that responsibility.

If you're a small practice, managing administration is a burden. As a single-practice doctor, you will likely need to merge with a larger practice at some point. That is the current evolution. Unfortunately, the larger practice says, "For us to make money, you need to see 15 or 20 patients a day." Scaling is how the larger practice covers the financial obligations of administrative management.

Instead of leading to an improvement in care, technology and innovation often become nothing more than an escalation of the existing, broken system. This is how we have arrived at the current state of modern medicine.

Culture Starts Internally

Culture sets the tone. It shapes performance, sparks ideas, fuels innovation, and gives people a sense of purpose. This is true in medicine, art, music, or any

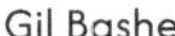

part of society; the common denominator is always people. When people are no longer at the center, culture inevitably begins to erode.

In the earlier decades of medicine, the 1950s, 1960s, and 1970s, the focus was unmistakably personal. Care centered around the physician, who knew patients by name, visited them in their homes, and was an integral part of the community. Television shows like Marcus Welby, M.D., that aired between 1969 and 1976, reflected this reality: the doctor with a black medical bag was trusted not just for expertise but for presence. Illness was addressed close to home, at the local hospital or community health center, not across the country at a distant institution.

Today, that doctor visit is rare. Medicine has become more procedural, transactional, and focused on documentation rather than connection. The black bag has been replaced by electronic medical records, prior authorizations, and complex billing codes. While science has advanced dramatically, the human bond between physician and patient, the very heartbeat of care, has been weakened. This erosion of culture is at the core of our current health system crisis.

Today, many institutions market it as, “Come to Istanbul for a hair transplant, and while you’re here, enjoy the city.” In such scenarios, the travel experience is designed to foster a doctor–patient connection. However, as healthcare shifts toward remote and high-tech delivery, we face new questions that extend far beyond the realm of medical tourism.

Robotic surgery, for example, enables doctors to operate on patients remotely, even when they are hundreds of miles away. This is a remarkable advance, especially for the nearly one in four Americans living in remote or rural communities. Yet technology only solves part of the problem. Who makes the diagnosis? Who secures approval from the insurer, Medicaid, or Medicare? Too often, those answers remain hidden in a black box.

This is why the culture of medicine must be revisited and strengthened. The more we hand control over to technology, the easier it is to forget that medicine exists for people, both those in need of healing and the clinicians offering care. No algorithm, robot, or large language model can replace the human responsibility to decide, listen, and act with empathy.

Calling AI "Artificial Intelligence" might be a misnomer in the context of medicine. Labeling AI as "Augmented Implementation" in a medical setting might be more appropriate. People are uncomfortable with a computerized intellect making life-and-death decisions about serious illnesses. There is an understandable reluctance for people to ask "Alexa" or "Siri" whether they should choose palliative care or endure another round of treatment.

My daughter came into our lives through the miracle of medical technology. Today, she is an award-winning author and social worker, directing her talents to inspire and help others.

This success did not come immediately. We were fortunate. Our insurance plan provided coverage, and we had a compassionate fertility specialist who treated us as partners in the process. What about families who lack that kind of support or coverage? These are deeply personal decisions that should remain between the family and the infertility specialist. Quality of life is not something for algorithms or robots to decide.

The voice and well-being of the clinician are essential. Data show that an inspired physician, who is passionate about the healing process, does more for their patients than one who is not. I've been blessed to have met such physicians. They are extraordinary people.

Sometimes, you will find a physician who has terrible bedside manner but is an outstanding clinician. However, superstars have great bedside manner and are also excellent physicians, producing great outcomes.

In my 2025 articles on empathy in the health setting on Medika Life, I refer to several such medical professionals. Their outcomes and patient satisfaction scores correspond to the strength of their empathy indicators. They are great at connecting with their patients and explaining the process.

Interestingly, if you study their patient satisfaction and outcome scores, they are disproportionately better than the cohort. Why? Their patients feel more connected, confident, and heard, and they organize their offices to better advocate for their patients.

One of the doctors I mentioned was having a lot of trouble with my insurance company, and he knew he was right. He and his office staff dedicated considerable time to staying on the phone with the insurance company and engaging with the system to explain why the payer was not doing its best to address their patients' needs.

An inspired and empathetic physician champions their patients in this fragmented system of care. They help the patient navigate the fragmentation because they see the patient not as an economic resource, but as a human being with concerns for which they can advocate. They know the patient through the lens of their desire to heal. They understand that managing the system has become an integral part of the process.

The concepts of effectiveness, efficiency, and empathy are essential to me. They should also be to you, whether you're a payer, product innovator, policymaker, or provider. They are a given if you're a patient, and we're all patients at some point.

This perspective has guided my work. Through the years, many people have reached out to me for guidance. In some cases, I have been able to connect them with physicians who are not only outstanding clinicians but also extraordinary healers. There is a difference between the two, and it is that difference, the human dimension, that ultimately saves lives.

I have been fortunate to be recognized as a top health tech influencer and health communicator, but I do not see that as an endpoint. For me, these moments remind me how much more there is to learn and apply. I have always been an early adopter. When Apple introduced its first connected device, the "Apple Newton", I bought one right off the production line. Yet, I have never

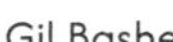

viewed technology as a replacement for people; I see it as an extension of our ability to connect and care.

In my experience, technology is most powerful when it amplifies the human dimension rather than overshadowing it. No algorithm, device, or platform can replace empathy. Purpose and connection must remain at the center, with technology as a tool to extend their reach.

To be a great clinician, you must possess excellent knowledge and genuinely care about applying that knowledge. Great clinicians with great empathy and a passion for healing are exponentially better healers because they genuinely want to engage in the healing process.

Those with excellent knowledge could be great bench scientists or pathologists. They may want to ponder the molecules of science. Simply having a PhD or MD does not necessarily make one a great healer, any more than it makes a healer great. You need both wisdom and caring to be a great healer.

What is the purpose of medicine? It is to make sick people feel better, sustain lives, and promote overall health. The system's role, in theory, is to do the same. The role of the payer is to achieve those same health outcomes in an economically, efficient, and effective manner. It is not to spare people from death, but to sustain and save life. The system must put people at the center of its operational model, not in isolation. People must be connected to, not isolated from, a comprehensive balance sheet that unites people and purpose.

When inner-city hospitals cannot pay salaries or keep the lights on, care breaks down. When people feel dismissed, they tend to disengage, delay care, become sicker, and ultimately incur higher costs. This is not just a matter of morality; it is also an economic issue.

Equally important is the respect and time given to health professionals. A system that squeezes every minute out of physicians, nurses, and allied health teams can lead to burnout, turnover, and a decline in the quality of care. When clinicians are exhausted and unsupported, the human connection with patients erodes, and no amount of technology or billing efficiency can replace it.

That is why patient satisfaction, experience, and engagement cannot be afterthoughts or tertiary priorities. They must sit at the center of the health system's design. Only when humanity shares equal weight with economics, and only when professionals are given the time and respect they need to do their best work, can we create an effective, efficient, and empathetic system. This shift, from fragmented transactions to coordinated, people-centered care, is not only the bridge to what comes next; it is the foundation of a truly sustainable health system.

Chapter 4

THE DATA PROBLEM: WHEN PEOPLE AND SYSTEMS DON'T TALK TO EACH OTHER

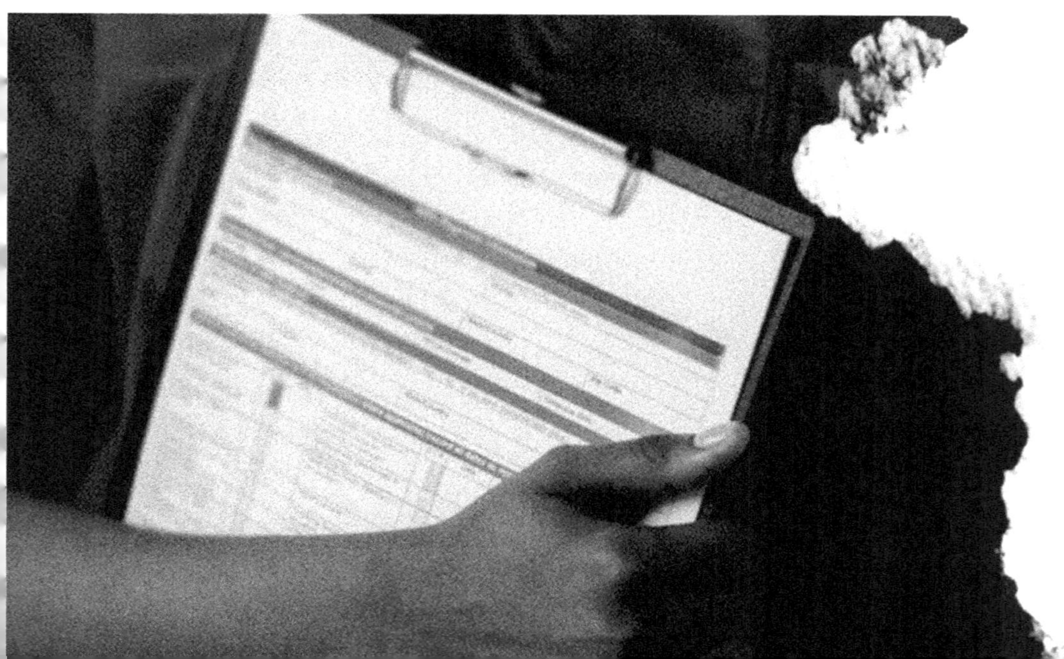

THE real challenge in our health system is not a shortage of resources; it is how effectively we make those resources available to those who need them.

Consider the numbers: When a nation spends 18.7 percent of its gross domestic product on health, as the U.S. does, according to the 2023 Centers for Medicare & Medicaid Services' National Health Expenditure Accounts, it must confront the hard truth that extraordinary investment has not translated into equitable or efficient care. It signals that nearly one-fifth of the nation's economic output is already dedicated to the well-being of its people. On paper, this should translate to timely, effective care that yields positive outcomes.

Unfortunately, that is not the reality. Despite leading the world in spending, the U.S. lags behind peer nations in basic measures of health. According to recent

CDC data, Americans today live on average 78.4 years, nearly four years shorter than the average of 82.5 years in other wealthy countries. The U.S. also reports an infant mortality rate of 5.4 deaths per 1,000 live births and a maternal mortality rate that is more than three times higher than in most developed nations. These outcomes underscore the paradox: extraordinary investment with results that fall short.

The U.S. and many European countries, including the United Kingdom and Germany, allocate a significant portion of their GDP to healthcare. The issue is not scarcity. The developed world has more than enough money to provide better services for its own people and even to support others globally. In the United States alone, we invest billions to train world-class physicians, nurses, and allied health professionals. This talent is sought after not only here but also in countries such as Hungary, Japan, India, and the UK. The problem is not the caliber of people or the level of spending. The problem lies in how poorly the system channels those investments toward those who need care the most.

Here lies the paradox: despite our abundant resources, illness still slips through the armor of money.

In the United States, a sedentary lifestyle and limited access to nutritious food have made obesity and related conditions rampant. These issues open the door to a cascade of non-communicable diseases such as diabetes, cardiovascular disease, and certain cancers, which are, tellingly, less common in many emerging nations. They are sometimes described as "diseases of wealth" because affluence often leads to more calorie-dense diets, a greater reliance on cars, increased screen time, and less daily physical activity. Wealth has not protected us; in some cases, it has made us more vulnerable.

Layered onto this abundance of medical challenges is another kind of abundance: information. We are awash in "big data." Sometimes it illuminates patterns and guides decisions; other times, it overwhelms or misleads. Long before today's debates about AI or electronic medical records, I confronted this tension firsthand—the challenge of transforming raw data, endless lab results, imaging scans, and billing codes into knowledge that clinicians and patients can actually act upon.

I learned this lesson as a graduate student in government affairs, lugging boxes of mainframe computer punch cards. At the time, this was the 1970s version of data storage across campuses and industry. What we now call "machine learning" was then a novel concept: feeding data into a program and letting it perform the intellectual heavy lifting. In the 1970s, that was a revolutionary development. Today, we'd call it "augmented intelligence," a way of extending human capacity, not replacing it.

Fast forward to our era of AI, GenAI, and large language models (LLMs), and the flood of information feels endless. Saul Wurman, the visionary behind TED and TEDMED, warned us in Information Anxiety that abundance can create paralysis. He was right. Data is finite, imperfect, and collected by fallible humans. It may come from our best intentions, but it is never flawless. Bad data leads to bad interpretations, compounded by human error. Yet for all its flaws, data remains the best path we have to see patterns, learn, and act.

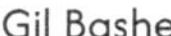

Ultimately, the core issue is how we access accurate medical information and how effectively we utilize it. Our tools for managing health data are advancing rapidly, but they still need a guiding philosophy to ensure they serve clinicians and patients well.

The answer is not more money. It is not more CME credits. It is not drowning clinicians in even larger streams of information.

The answer lies in stepping back and recognizing the human dimension of healing, including our mindset, emotions, and capacity for empathy. It creates space for humanity to be present in every encounter and decision. We have neglected this human dimension, despite it being the most critical element of care.

Listen to the daily news about healthcare, and what do you hear? Economics and policy. Obesity. Budgets. Social inequities. Costs of drugs and devices. Prior authorizations. These are real issues, but they swirl around the patient rather than touching the core.

The real questions are simpler and more urgent: Can this 55-year-old woman return to health? Can this child with asthma breathe easier? Can this man lower his BMI, cholesterol, and A1C before it is too late? These are the questions at the heart of health system kinetics, whether the system's energy is aligned toward restoring people or solely directed to sustaining itself.

We spend endless hours debating the periphery while neglecting the core: people. We study the human body but forget its soul—and not just the patient's soul, but also the humanity of the CEO, the CFO, the chief science officer, the senator on the health committee, and the leaders at Health and Human Services (HHS), the Food and Drug Administration (FDA), Centers for Medicare & Medicaid Services (CMS), and the National Health Service (NHS).

The narrative must shift. It cannot be about the "it." It must be about the "us."

The Cost of Disconnection

At the center of the struggle to use data effectively for patients is not a lack of information, but the way it is scattered and siloed. Fragmentation is the fault line running through American healthcare.

For patients, fragmentation is not an abstract concept; it is a lived reality. Many people see multiple doctors across different systems and specialties, none of whom know each other. My own gastroenterologist and cardiologist, for instance, are unaware of each other's existence. Each knows only what we discuss in the exam room. However, their work is deeply connected. My cardiology history could shape my gastroenterologist's decisions during a routine colonoscopy. If I experienced a gastrointestinal bleed, those details could inform my cardiologist's care. When the system keeps them siloed, the patient becomes the only connector.

The data from these encounters eventually become part of an electronic medical record (EMR). In theory, that record should be the common thread. This navigational tool could enable each doctor to see the entire picture and make informed decisions. Yet, in practice, EMRs are often incomplete, inconsistent, or inaccessible across different systems. Interoperability remains a promise, not a reality. What is missing isn't

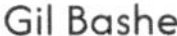

just the data; it's the focus on me, the person behind the numbers.

EMRs are riddled with mistakes. Just check your medication list. Drugs you stopped years ago still appear because they were pulled in automatically from another database. Every practice has to delete them manually at each visit. Your outdated medical history follows you from doctor to doctor.

This is the deeper truth: EMR data is derived from people. It is their lives, their symptoms, their experiences. When the system treats data as an end in itself, it erases the very humanity that gives the numbers meaning.

That truth shows up in the doctors themselves. I know exceptional physicians who understand human experience, physicians who pause, connect, listen, and treat patients as individuals. Still, I know others who, pressed by time and systemic pressures, engage poorly, reducing encounters to transactions. Fragmentation doesn't just divide our data; it divides our humanity.

One patient once told me that after waiting weeks for an appointment, their physician barely looked up from the computer, asked only a few rushed questions, and ended the visit in under five minutes. That is what it feels like when care becomes a transaction instead of a relationship.

Dr. Alison Grann reminds her team, "I want my staff to treat patients as I would want to be treated." It's a simple but effective equation. Who wants to be dismissed, disregarded, or diminished?

Why do these outstanding doctors provide counsel and care that patients consider exceptional, and why are exceptional patient experiences the exception instead of the rule? It's not because we structure the medical industry to disregard patient experience. As I have pointed out, some doctors are global role models who have structured their lives, positions, and departments to think and act as they do, yet operate under the same system as those who perform poorly.

Medical students must master the fundamentals of physiology, chemistry, and biology. Science and specialization are essential. However, if training ends there, we have failed. Future physicians must also learn the psychology of care: fear in an anxious patient, the confusion of someone sifting through misinformation, the courage of a person searching for hope. They need to understand how to mobilize the system, not just to treat disease, but to comfort the person who carries it.

The ability to interpret information wisely is a crucial aspect of the medical profession. It is not about knowing everything; it is about understanding what matters. Medical schools rarely teach this skill, yet it is one of the most critical qualities we should look for when selecting tomorrow's doctors. A doctor can treat a patient according to their specialty. However, who will treat the person?

I first met Dr. Jerry Groopman of Harvard Medical School in the mid-1980s at a press briefing held at the Pierre Hotel in New York City, where the first biotherapeutic for cancer treatment was being discussed. Author of How Doctors Think, Dr. Groopman later discovered in 2007 an important truth in his practice: patients with a faith-based background often fared better through illness than those without. He explained, "I started out as an agnostic or atheist, and from the patients who have faith, I re-found my faith." Their spirituality gave him an avenue to connect with them, reminding him that medicine is not only about science, but also about meaning.

The best physicians never forget this. When they examine a person with an illness, they see an individual first and foremost, not a diagnosis code.

I say this as someone who is an avid technology advocate. Yet in every message, program, and conversation, I remind myself that I am not engaging with data points; I am communicating with people, their thoughts, opinions, and hopes. That mindset makes the difference between a transaction and a connection.

This tension between data and empathy is not abstract; it has reached into my own family. My daughter once visited a highly recommended physician. When she described her symptoms, the surgeon dismissed her account, trusting his knowledge over her lived experience. I was stunned by his comment, “Who are you going to believe, another patient or me?” That response did not sit right with me. Isn’t the patient’s learned experience worth something? In her case, it was worth its weight in gold.

Afterward, we saw another robotic surgeon who validated the patient experience. This second doctor was empathetic and a clear communicator. He saw the clinical data and considered the patient’s condition. The surgery was precise, and the results were almost immediate and life-changing.

When my daughter met with the first robotic surgeon, her weight was in the high 80s. If she had chosen to be treated by this doctor, she might have eventually needed an IV TPN feeding line. Conversely, with the second surgeon, she was able to begin eating well, without pain from a compressed artery, and her weight eventually rebounded.

The second surgeon was also considered one of the best robotic surgeons in the country, but he was not chosen solely on the basis of his clinical skills. He was selected because he believed in and highlighted both the patient experience and the data.

Using your imagination requires you to think outside the box. The first doctor remained in the box, fixated on what he knew, while the second one considered the patient's journey, the terror of what lay ahead, and the pain of losing hope.

The second surgeon provided the patient and us, the caregivers, with an incredibly positive and hopeful experience. An individual doctor can make or break the patient's and their family's health and mental health experience.

Health Data Without Context

Information is most valuable when it can be applied accurately and effectively. The democratization of data is not a technical exercise. It is the foundation of trust. At its core, it means relaying accurate information so people can make informed choices. True democracy thrives when everyone has access to correct data to guide reasonable decisions. Health is no different.

Physicians and health professionals must have access to accurate information, and just as important, they must have the time to verify it. Is this the correct data for the right patient at the right time? Even patients

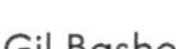

and families often read the hospital chart after a visit to catch errors and ensure accuracy.

The problem is that our system was never designed to guarantee this accuracy. Inaccuracies slip into medical records and, over time, harden into "facts." A patient once told me her chart listed her as a smoker, though she had never smoked a day in her life. Despite correcting it multiple times, the error reappeared at every visit, affecting how clinicians interacted with her and even influencing the tests that were ordered. These distortions become part of a person's medical history, replicated again and again. That is not democratization; that is institutionalized error.

On the other end of the spectrum, some doctors become defensive when patients come in informed and seek to engage in peer-like conversation. Yet shutting down those discussions only widens the gap. The opposite of data democratization is misinformation, and once misinformation takes root, trust evaporates. Without trust, the system collapses under the weight of its own contradictions.

This danger is not hypothetical. During the COVID-19 pandemic, we saw how misinformation and rumors about vaccines, treatments, and even the basic science of transmission spread faster than the virus itself. Life was lost not only to disease but also due to eroded trust. That mistrust has carried forward to vaccines that have been demonstrated to spare lives from once-conquered viruses. The same is true in today's digital era, where AI systems can "hallucinate" facts that look authoritative but are dangerously wrong.

If caregivers provide a doctor with misinformation, whether intentionally or unintentionally, they create a ripple of falsehood that can distort care. Perhaps they misunderstood the patient, perhaps they shaded the truth, or perhaps they repeated something inaccurate. Whatever the cause, the result is the same: the system becomes a conduit for misinformation, not a guardian of truth.

What do we trust? Do we trust what is written in a medical record? Do we trust what we read online, even though so much of it turns out to be misinformation? It is human nature to believe what we see or hear, whether it comes from a chart or an influencer's post. That instinct makes trust powerful and dangerous when the source is wrong.

I've seen this personally. More than once, my wife or I have had to advocate for an electronic medical record correction. Once the audio transcription system mistakenly merged my father-in-law's medical history into my mother-in-law's file, suddenly attributing his cancer diagnosis to her EMR. If that error were embedded in the system, it would become her "truth." Yet, it also happened in the "old days" when doctors scribbled notes into charts.

The implications are immediate and lasting. Medical treatment plans can be accidentally distorted. In another case, the ability to obtain life or long-term care insurance was jeopardized. The middle-aged patient's history of one to ten fainting episodes over his life became 110! Instead of fixing the mistake, the doctor dug in his heels. He preferred an institutionalized error to admitting he was wrong. That is not data democratization; that is betrayal.

How can we achieve the democratization of data? How can the machine distinguish the accurate from the inaccurate? It can't. The information, good or bad, originates from people. Remember, all information, such as that from my punch cards from the 1970s, derives from human beings. We often overlook this aspect when it comes to medical information systems.

How can we make people care about accurate medical information? To begin, we need to encourage people to prioritize the accuracy of information. If people no longer feel motivated to go the extra mile, or if the healer-patient relationship weakens, who will still care about EMR accuracy? The accuracy of that information has a domino effect, from long-term care to life insurance. People fear that this information will be used against them in the short or long term.

Patients rarely have equal decision-making power. The real levers of authority belong to the system's two engines: the innovators who develop new science and therapies, and the providers who deliver them. These groups push the system forward. Yet, if progress is not centered on people and their experiences, then the momentum is wasted.

Of course, information can be streamlined in countless ways with AI, augmented intelligence, and large language models. Still, technology alone will not democratize data. That requires something deeper: the will to do right by the people the health sector is meant to serve.

So, ask yourself: as a provider, policymaker, or innovator, are you doing right by your patients? Are you fulfilling your calling? The Hippocratic Oath reminds us to do no harm. That principle must apply not only to treatments and procedures but also to the information we record, share, and rely on. Inaccurate data is its own form of harm. Accuracy is not optional; it is an ethical imperative.

In all applications of innovation, technology, and information, we must ask ourselves a key question: are they being deployed in a way that minimizes harm and maximizes benefit?

Depth of Engagement

Clinical guidelines are designed for the average patient, not the individual. Doctors are trained to look for the herd of horses, not the lone zebra.

This is not caused by providers wishing to ignore personal needs. It happens because their performance is measured against regulatory and systemic standards—metrics that evaluate whether a molecule, drug, or device works in the abstract human body, not in this patient's life. Pharmaceuticals are judged the same way: did the product help or harm the average body, not how it fits the daily reality of one person.

The disconnect widens because pharmaceutical and medical device companies rarely sit down with payers to ask a critical question: how do we get this product quickly to the people who will benefit most? Too often, products already proven in practice are labeled "experimental" to avoid cost or disruption. I lived this with my own child when a capsule endoscopy, the so-called "smart camera pill," was dismissed as experimental by the payer despite two decades of clinical use and thousands of successful outcomes.

For payers, the focus remains a system of financial checks and balances. The priority is cost management, not the patient's lived experience (or a child's comfort). However, what if we reframed the question? Instead of asking only whether a cheaper product is "good enough," we should also ask: good enough for whom? For some, a less expensive option may suffice. For others, lifestyle factors, such as needing fewer pills a day, make a different product the better choice, even life-sustaining.

Guidelines and systems help define the composite picture of health. However, people are not composites. They are individuals with unique lives, priorities, and needs, and they deserve to be treated that way.

The complexity of treatment is something I have experienced myself. Not long ago, to quell a bout of bronchitis, I had several prescriptions that required taking pills multiple times a day at different hours. That kind of regimen would challenge almost anyone. Now imagine facing it without the support of organizational skills, a family, or a caregiver. Recovery would slow or fail entirely. Yet payers rarely stop to consider whether fewer pills or a simpler regimen might save a life. They largely see cost.

There was a time when doctors could step in. Your physician once had the freedom to decide how to treat you based on what they knew about you as a person. That freedom has been stripped away, replaced by a payer's need to manage costs across millions of patients. The system no longer sees you; it sees only averages.

Could AI and predictive modeling be used to reverse this trend? Could it tailor treatments to patient types, lifestyles, and circumstances? The information is here. What is missing is accuracy, application, and the will to use data in the service of individuals rather than institutions.

We live in an age of breathtaking innovation. New technologies, regulatory approvals, and ever-rising spending have transformed what is possible. Yet many hospitals in the U.S. are still barely breaking even. Chronic diseases climb unchecked. Obesity morphs into a national epidemic. We are advancing technologically, but not medically. We are seeing the rise of innovation and the fall of empathy.

We cannot shrug and say, "The system is too big to change." We must not stand idle. The human dynamic must be restored to the center of health. We must return to the calling that drew so many into medicine in the first place—not simply to fight disease, but to serve people.

Doctors and nurses must be supported throughout their professional journey to stay faithful to their calling: "I want to heal people. I want innovative medicines that improve people's health. I want to ensure that people have access to the medical treatment that makes sense."

Many of the health sector's issues stem from the fact that treating disease is expensive. However, treating disease should not be our baseline. Our baseline should be preventing and curing disease. People want to live long, happy lives, but that is not our focus right now.

To elaborate, consider a child with regularly scheduled medical checkups. These routine checkups seem to be an inherent part of the medical structure for younger people, but why not for older adults? Why don't 75-year-olds undergo mandatory hearing or eyesight exams to reduce cognitive decline? It's because the school system often covers the cost of children's checkups. If you're 75 and need a hearing aid, you usually have to pay for it.

There is an adage that says, "He who writes the rules, rules!" Consider the absurd rules that govern our healthcare system and senior care. Medicare still doesn't cover refractions for my 93-year-old mother-in-law, so she has to pay out-of-pocket for that part of the eye exam that checks how the eyes focus light. Despite a clear link between vision and falls, which she has had, no coverage is given.

Now, both poor vision and poor hearing also contribute to dementia. What is the cost of a broken hip repair versus a hearing aid? The average cost of an inpatient hip replacement is $30,700. The average cost of prescription-model hearing aids ranges from $2,100 to $3,300 per pair.

Pharmaceutical and product innovation companies are judged relentlessly by investors, stakeholders, employees, and regulators. Their mandate is not measured in lives touched, but in profits delivered. Success, in the current model, is defined by shareholder dividends and stock performance. Patients, meanwhile, are absent from the balance sheet.

In today's biopharma system, success is narrowly measured by whether a drug meets regulatory requirements.

Is it safe? Is it effective? Once those boxes are ticked, the next bar to be cleared is sales. Yet, nowhere in investor briefings and quarterly earnings calls is there a PowerPoint slide for patient satisfaction, equitable access, or whether the right person received the right drug at the right time. The real question, rarely asked, is how we reconcile the return on investment that shareholders demand with the public health outcomes society urgently needs.

I've lived the gap myself. When a payer denied me a medication, my doctor spent an extra hour on the phone arguing, sending documentation, and waiting for an answer. No one reimbursed her for that time. She carried the burden because she chose to advocate for me. Many doctors cannot afford to spend that kind of time, and so they yield. That is why private practice primary care is vanishing; the economics punish advocacy.

Not every physician will fight the system. Why would they? They are not compensated for resistance. Their performance is measured against system profitability, not their willingness to champion individual patients. In many cases, the only advocate left is the patient, a family member, or the rare health provider unwilling to surrender.

The greatest frustration for patients is not just the denial of a product or service. It is the gauntlet of roadblocks—the endless delays, appeals, and opaque information—that keep physicians from quickly grasping the arc of a patient's medical journey or seeing the best standard of care delivered.

Technology has the potential to shift this balance. Yet this will happen only if it amplifies human understanding, empathy, and access, not if it becomes another instrument of efficiency divorced from people. Investors, policymakers, and providers must recognize that the strongest return on investment is measured not only in quarterly earnings, but in lives extended, suffering reduced, and trust restored. That is the ROI that sustains both business and society.

Physician-Guided Digital Health Experiences

We're all fascinated by AI. The capabilities of large language models are impressive. Yet, while we sprint ahead with health tech innovation, we often overlook the element that gives health its soul: empathy.

Some of the most helpful and even "empathetic" digital features now available are those that give patients real-time insight into their health. I use a device from AliveCor. By placing my thumbs on the device and opening the app on my phone, I can generate a six-lead electrocardiogram of my heart. Although I don't have a heart condition, I'm fascinated by medical technology and proactively interested in my health. It enables me to monitor my heart function and, if necessary, share the results with my doctor.

This is democratization of information in action: producing medical data that I, as a patient, can interpret and choose to share. Yet, here lies the dilemma: will that data be used for me or against me?

On the positive side, this information could strengthen compliance with treatment, confirm heart health, and accelerate lifesaving interventions. In the wrong hands, it could be turned against me, to label me with a "pre-existing condition," to raise my premiums, or even to deny life or long-term care insurance. In such a system, knowledge becomes a liability. Who would want to be proactive if that very curiosity could be weaponized against them?

This paradox demands executive reflection. Technology companies, payers, and policymakers cannot simply marvel at their ability to generate data. They must commit to ensuring that data empowers individuals rather than punishes them. Otherwise, we risk creating a world where taking responsibility for your health becomes a disadvantage.

Data without solutions is just more noise. That is why we must double down on the human dynamic in medicine. The goal is to provide patients with more information and give them the confidence, support, and protection they need to use that information without fear. If executives, innovators, and policymakers want to win trust, they must treat democratized information as a public good, never as a pretext to deny care.

Some policymakers of government agencies, particularly at the staff level, are incredibly passionate and imaginative public servants. Several of them earn far less than they would in the private sector. They are also required to act within the parameters of the law. Laws concerning the medical system are passed by Congress and signed by the president, but implemented by these public servants. These are individuals guided by science and regulatory law in developing tools or determining how to accomplish a task more efficiently, but only to the extent permitted by law. The next step is integrating collaboration to improve the human condition.

That's the bottleneck. That's where everything breaks down. It's not a failure of imagination; it's a failure of connection. People operate within narrow parameters, each holding only part of the puzzle. You can't see the full picture without the missing pieces, scattered across specialties, systems, and organizations. You can't imagine what's possible because you're not allowed to see it.

We continually add new tools, including AI and large language models, believing that faster processing will solve the problem. Yet, speed is not the answer. Information without human interpretation remains noise.

Action must begin with accuracy. Data must move through the system efficiently, be clearly collected, communicated openly, and received in a manner that makes sense. Only then can it be assessed and used wisely by the next person in the chain of care.

Communication can be the linchpin. A doctor should feel free to say, "I want to check some of the information in your report to make sure it's accurate." Too often, they don't. It's not because doctors, nurses, or pharmacists don't care; the system has stripped away their two most precious resources: time and permission.

Health professionals today face a mountain of data. They lack the breathing room to pause, question, and verify. They are trained to assume that what's in the EMR is correct, even when experience tells them it may not be. In a culture that rewards efficiency over accuracy, few feel free to admit uncertainty and utter the most human words: "I don't know, let me check."

It always comes back to the human dynamic: empathy, curiosity, collaboration, and the willingness to see beyond the screen to reconnect with the person in front of us. We lean too heavily on technology when the system truly needs a human touch.

The various components of the health sector, including pharma, payers, providers, innovators, and policymakers, must come together around a shared purpose. This purpose is not simply to generate more data or design the next device, but to make information accurate, accessible, and meaningful in individuals' lives.

If we remove that purpose, we strip health of its social impact and reduce the system to a heartless machine. That is not the future any of us, investors, executives, clinicians, or patients, should accept.

Everything—money, talent, innovation, technology, science, molecules, and devices—exists for one reason: to serve humanity. The test before us is whether we will have the courage and imagination to make it so.

Chapter 5

THE PREVENTION GAP: WHY WE SPEND ON SICKNESS, NOT HEALTH

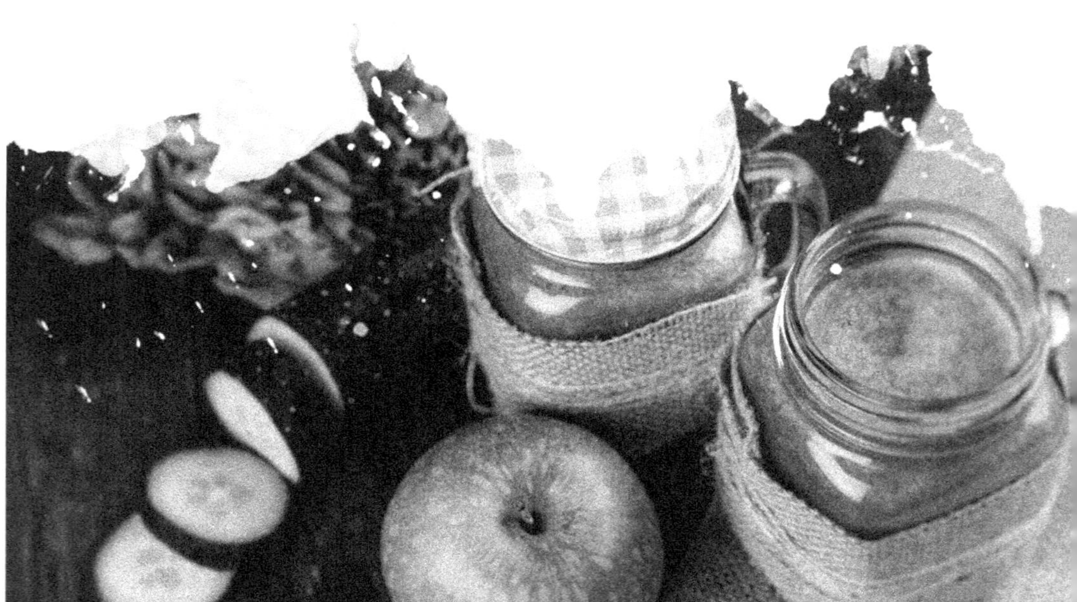

In the wake of Brian Thompson's tragic murder, the insurance industry's disconnect from the people it serves became painfully visible. Instead of uniting in grief, some public reactions pivoted toward anger and frustration with the system itself. The fact that expressions of rage surfaced alongside news of his death should have been a wake-up call: trust had eroded so deeply that even tragedy was filtered through resentment toward the industry.

While we might expect insurers to have learned that greater transparency and truthfulness were urgently needed, business has continued much the same. This is not out of malice but out of a model that too often feels tone-deaf to the people it serves. What might be called an "Insurance Shell Game" shifts the burden of costs away from payers and onto the very people they are meant to protect, leaving nearly one in five

American adults carrying medical debt. In 2022, the Kaiser Family Foundation reported that this burden now exceeds $220 billion nationwide.

The result is a system in which people pay for insurance yet still shoulder much of the cost of their care. Premiums continue to skyrocket. Under such conditions, frustration is inevitable. Leaders at the C-suite level would do well to pause and ask themselves, “If I were the consumer, how would I feel realizing I was both insured and still paying heavily out of pocket?” The answer is clear: furious, hurt, and frightened. Too often, that perspective is absent from decision-making.

What erodes most in this dynamic is not money but care itself. Empathy dries up when the system reduces medicine to transactions, processes, and technologies. Yet caring remains the heartbeat of healing, the essence of why medicine exists. Rebuilding trust begins with centering on that truth.

Scripture serves as a reminder of the patient’s urgent need for health. When Moses learned that his sister Miriam was ill with leprosy, he prayed the simplest of prayers, “God, please heal her now.” In its brevity, it carried the full weight of compassion and immediacy. Healing requires more than protocols or payments; it calls upon the deepest part of our humanity.

My desire to support people facing health challenges comes from the imprint of my own journey. I have witnessed kindness and the healing strength it brings. I have also seen horror and the scars it leaves behind. These experiences remind me that when people are ill, they are anxious, uncertain, and afraid. How we respond can either ease or intensify that burden.

When a health system loses its sense of caring, it shrinks into mere transactions, focused on money earned rather than lives supported. Only empathy at the center allows it to fulfill its greater purpose.

That lesson is not confined to hospitals or clinics. It plays out in our daily encounters. Walking through the streets of New York City, I sometimes carry small bills to offer when asked, but more importantly, I pause to say "hello." The true gift is not the money. It is an acknowledgment, a chance to restore dignity, even if only briefly.

A younger colleague once asked me, "Why do you do that? Aren't you just encouraging them to beg?" The question missed the point. What matters is not the transaction but the connection. The same is true in medicine: without connection, there can be no true healing.

People often reach a point of desperation when they no longer see options. In those moments, even a small gesture can signal, "You are seen. You matter." If that act helps them feed a family member or care for a pet, it may spark enough hope to carry them forward. That spark is what our health system must learn to ignite, not through charity but through a culture of empathy and connection that treats every person as worthy of being seen.

I approach people proactively because asking for help carries the risk of humiliation. After hundreds of rejections, a kind word or gesture can restore someone's dignity. Even more important is trust. If I don't have cash and promise to return with something else, I make sure I come back. For many people in that position, opportunities to experience trust are rare.

Patients in today's health system face a similar scarcity of trust. They pay premiums, deductibles, and copays, yet too often find themselves waiting months for approval of the treatments their doctors have recommended. In fact, a 2022 American Medical Association survey found that 94 percent of physicians reported experiencing care delays due to prior authorization. One-third stated that it had led to a serious adverse event for a patient. For patients, it can feel like standing on a street corner, hat in hand, hoping the system will notice them.

That is not sustainable. Health cannot be built on a framework of winners and losers. It must be built on empathy and collaboration, where every participant: payers, providers, innovators, and policymakers, recognizes that we all win when people feel cared for, as if that truly matters to everyone involved. Remember the urgency of Moses, upon seeing his sister's suffering, who utters the shortest prayer in the Bible. That urgency and compassion speak to the humanity our system must embrace.

Technology is one of humanity's greatest tools, born of our ingenuity and drive to improve life. In health, its purpose is not to replace kindness or connection but to extend our reach, sharpen our insights, and make us more effective in caring for one another.

Some say the stethoscope was medicine's first great innovation. I believe the true first innovation was bedside manner, the healer's ability to listen, comfort, and connect. The stethoscope strengthened that connection by giving physicians a new way to hear what was happening inside the body, but it never replaced the act of listening to the person. The lesson is clear: technology should enhance humanity, not eclipse it.

That same principle must guide us today. Innovation is essential, but innovation for its own sake is not enough. The true promise of health technology lies in its ability to help people live longer, healthier, and more sustainable lives. That truth must remain at the center of every decision, whether we are payers, product innovators, policymakers, or providers.

Artificial intelligence, for example, is already helping clinicians diagnose more quickly and even capture in-room conversations to create patient notes. Yet here is the risk: if the time saved by AI is redirected solely toward efficiency, it will result in shorter visits and less connection, not more. The opportunity lies in using that time to deepen effectiveness, giving patients more attention, listening, and empathy that the system too often squeezes out.

Real change will require a fundamentally different approach that moves beyond incremental fixes, confronts the system's contradictions, and rebuilds healthcare around both profits and people.

Sick Care vs. Health Care

Achieving positive health outcomes has only highlighted the stark economic divide that Americans experience. If someone is fortunate to have the means to join a health club, hire a personal trainer, or purchase low-sugar, low-calorie foods, they are more likely to maintain a healthier path. If they are economically challenged and need to feed their family, a steady diet of carbs and fast food is more likely to be on their menu because it's affordable and easily obtained between work shifts.

Economic divides are not abstractions; they are visible even in childhood. At my father's gas station, located adjacent to an under-resourced neighborhood, he often fixed cars for free for families who couldn't afford repairs. He knew a family with many children and limited financial resources. Their car needed constant attention, and he understood they couldn't afford the repairs. So he worked on it for hours, and when they asked, "How much do we owe you?" he would wave it off. Even if they insisted, he'd say, "No, it's okay."

Life has given me a series of these "mini-movies," snapshots that reveal not just moments but patterns. Statistics come alive when you've seen them play out in real time. It isn't rocket science to recognize that a child who grows up without access to nutritious food will carry those effects for years. That is reality. When we disconnect those mini-movies from decisions about food assistance programs or Medicaid access, we turn our backs on both the problem and the people.

People don't want their cars simply patched; they want to know they can get safely and reliably from place to place. Health is no different.

Programs like Medicaid provide essential healthcare access for people with limited financial resources;

however, uneven reimbursement and gaps in provider participation often mean that care begins only after an illness has taken root. Medicare serves a different population and offers more consistent coverage, with broader acceptance among clinicians, but it was never designed to address the root causes of disease. These important programs expose the same systemic truth: in America, we treat sickness far more aggressively than we prevent it.

I grew up witnessing the consequences of poor nutrition firsthand. Our family income nudged us into the middle class, but not always far enough to absorb every risk. At my father's gas station, children would cross the street each morning to buy "breakfast" from vending machines: candy bars for 15 cents, soda for a quarter. Decades later, that memory has a darker meaning: in low-income areas, such choices are too often the only ones available, setting many children on paths toward obesity, heart disease, and diabetes.

For many of those same children who lived near the gas station, the only consistently healthy meal might have been a subsidized school lunch. According to USDA data, in 2023–2024, nearly 29.4 million children participated in the National School Lunch Program on an average school day, with 21.1 million receiving a free or reduced-price lunch. Even so, as budget cuts squeeze these programs, that safety net is fraying. The result is stark: the social determinants of health become an incubator for illness.

We have embedded sickness into society at a young age. Today, more than 136 million Americans live with some form of diabetes or prediabetes. In a nation of 350 million, that means more than one in

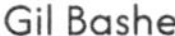

three people is touched by this epidemic. According to OECD data, Japan's obesity rate is about 4 percent compared to 43 percent in the U.S.

We have allowed obesity and its consequences to spread largely unchecked. These outcomes are not abstract; they stem from choices we make, or fail to make, about prevention, nutrition, and equity. Social determinants of health, poverty, food security, and unsafe neighborhoods can even switch on genetic predisposition, turning risk into disease.

Heart disease remains the leading killer of men and women worldwide, and certainly in the United States. We also know that heart disease, diabetes, and at least four major cancers are directly related to weight. The obesity epidemic has set off a cascade of non-communicable diseases, disproportionately claiming the lives of the most vulnerable.

Who are the most vulnerable? They are people living in communities where healthy food, quality care, and reliable health education are out of reach. Smoking, lack of access to nutritious foods, and limited opportunities for physical activity are not abstract risk factors; they are daily realities shaped by income, geography, and access.

In this way, we build sickness into the system. Whether by intention or neglect, the result is the same: people arrive at hospital doors already burdened by disease. Some have insurance and will receive care that gives them a chance to recover. Others lack coverage or resources, and their outcomes are predictably worse.

The divide is not random; it is preordained by the structure we have created.

At its core, we have designed a system centered more on economics than equity. Hospitals are asked to operate on razor-thin budgets, especially in rural communities. Physicians and health professionals shoulder the strain, forced to see more patients in less time, even as the complexity of care rises.

The imbalance extends to the workforce itself. The system undervalues primary care physicians, the very doctors who prevent illness and sustain long-term health. With crushing medical school debt and lower pay, fewer young doctors are choosing primary care. Over time, this shortage threatens to erode the frontline of medicine.

We have a system where doctors who want to enter primary care or internal medicine often struggle to pay off student loans and household expenses. Even as we bring in highly skilled professionals such as physician assistants and nurse practitioners, economics do not favor prevention. Because payer reimbursement is lower at the primary care level, more physicians are drawn toward higher-paying specialties. In fact, primary care doctors earn roughly half of what specialists earn. That gap steers talent away from the places we need it most, preventing disease rather than confronting sickness.

The Hidden Cost of Convenience

Clearly, we are not willing to invest in preventing the progression of illnesses that are waiting to strike. We invest heavily in treating diseases but not in preventing them in the first place.

If someone is living with excess weight, whether rooted in metabolism or circumstance, they are at higher risk for many complications, including heart disease and orthopedic problems. Data from one study indicate that 38.5 percent of patients undergoing total knee replacement were classified as having obesity, a finding highlighted by Thomas C. B. Dehn, MBBS, FRCS, in The Annals of the Royal College of Surgeons of England in 2007. This is not a trivial find. It serves as a reminder that weight is a complex medical and social issue shaped by biology, environment, stress, and household resources.

Yet, as a nation, we still have not united around a simple truth: allowing chronic conditions like this to advance unchecked is far more costly than engaging them in the first place. We know it has reached epidemic levels, and we add to the physical burden by adding layers of emotional baggage to medical complexities. Unfortunately, our current policies and reimbursement structures rarely reward health professionals for preventing illness; they are paid for treating it after the fact.

The same short-term thinking shows up in our approach to school meals. Instead of exploring how to utilize the lunch system to establish a pattern of healthy eating, budget constraints often prompt schools to opt for cheaper, calorie-dense foods that are high in starch and sugar. A 2023 USDA report found that more than 90 percent of schools struggle to meet updated nutrition standards because the options are more expensive. In the long run, these economic trade-offs fuel obesity, diabetes, and heart disease, conditions that are far more expensive to treat than to prevent.

The American public has been conditioned to consume sugar in excess of healthy limits. A sweet treat in moderation is not the problem; the problem is that sugar has quietly become embedded in daily routines, sprinkled on cereal, stirred into coffee, baked into snacks, and ending meals with dessert.

According to the Harvard School of Public Health, Americans consume an average of about 17 teaspoons of added sugar per day, nearly double the World Health Organization's recommended limit of six teaspoons. By comparison, adults in the United Kingdom average about twelve teaspoons, while in Japan, the average is closer to seven teaspoons. This relentless exposure makes sugar a prominent feature of the American diet and a driver of obesity, diabetes, and heart disease.

The more time-pressed we are, the less we prepare our own meals and the more we choose pre-prepared snacks instead. This is how an entire alternative to the "junk food" cottage industry has developed in response to the growing need to deliver meal ingredients directly to our doorsteps. During the COVID-19 pandemic, meal kit subscriptions provided nutritious options packaged for convenience. They worked well for those with the means to afford them. Again, economics shape access to health.

When fruits and vegetables are expensive, a family with four or five mouths to feed may not have the money for nutritious food. Carbohydrates are filling and inexpensive. Pasta, potatoes, and processed foods are tasty

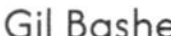

and cheap. It is no surprise, then, that according to the CDC, fewer than one in ten American adults eats the recommended daily servings of fruits and vegetables.

For many, the challenge is not just cost but access. Nearly 20 million Americans live in food deserts, communities where grocery stores and fresh produce are scarce, a reality reflected in USDA Economic Research Service data, which estimates that 18.8 million people reside in low-income, low-access census tracts.

The food label system we have "sells" us calories. A product may appear reasonable in calories, but that number hides the full story. It may also be loaded with sugar, sodium, saturated fats, or chemical additives that offer little nutritional value and, over time, harm health. One hundred calories may not sound like much, but if those calories come from a soda or a bag of chips rather than vegetables, fruit, or protein, the impact on the body is entirely different over time.

As a result, we are ingesting an increasing number of artificial additives and highly processed ingredients. While the body is made up of chemicals, not all substances interact with it in the same way. Diets high in added sugars, sodium, and trans fats can disrupt normal physiology, contributing to high blood pressure, elevated cholesterol levels, and increased blood sugar levels.

Where do we start the conversation on improved health outcomes for an entire nation? How do we invest in a way that stops the widespread progression of illness in our lives?

When I was a child, and even into the 1970s, most fruits and vegetables were available only in season. While international shipping and cold storage existed, they had not yet made fresh produce widely or affordably available year-round. Today, it is common to see cherries in winter or asparagus in summer, choices made possible by global transport and preservation technologies. These choices come with trade-offs that require us to consider cost, sustainability, and nutritional value.

Does this justify the way we have allowed a sick care system to dominate? Of course not. The real issue is not only a lack of fruits and vegetables, but also an economic framework that rewards low-cost, short-term fixes and incentivizes rejections of medical claims instead of prevention. Fragmentation unintentionally seeds sick care, leaving people treated only when they are ill rather than supported to stay well.

This is where President Lyndon B. Johnson, the architect of "The Great Society" and a champion of Medicare and Medicaid, sought to bridge policy, people, and potential. His vision was clear. The sick should not be impoverished simply because they were sick. As Johnson declared at the signing of Medicare: "No longer will illness crush and destroy the savings that they have so carefully put away over a lifetime so that they might enjoy dignity in their later years." Health, in his view, was a matter of dignity as much as survival.

We have drifted from that clarity. Consider how schools, once a frontline of prevention, have steadily seen their budgets cut. Physical education was never a luxury; it was a foundation of long-term health.

Children had recess, playgrounds, and after-school sports that kept bodies moving and minds alert. One by one, these opportunities have been stripped away as priorities shifted and public funds evaporated.

A healthy body supports a healthy mind. Schools that provide balanced meals and physical education are not just educating; they are building resilience against future illness. Some professionals suggest that both contribute to children's well-being, including mental health. Yet, over time, prevention has slipped down the list of priorities, and the very places that could teach lifelong health habits have been undermined by budget cuts.

If fragmentation has led us astray, empathy and collaboration can guide us back. When policymakers, educators, and health leaders ask, "How would this decision affect my child, my parent, my community?" they begin to reshape practice with humanity at the center. Empathy and collaboration do not replace innovation or profit; they give them purpose.

Skeptics argue that taxpayer dollars should not be used to fund gym class or after-school sports, or that nutritious lunches are a luxury. However, the truth is the opposite. Every dollar cut from school nutrition or physical activity programs is not a savings, but a deferred cost that society pays later in the form of higher rates of obesity, diabetes, and other chronic diseases. Children's health is not an optional expense; it is a down payment on the nation's health.

We rightly emphasize math, science, history, and English, but how much of our education is dedicated to keeping our bodies healthy and alive? Very little. In an age when artificial intelligence can provide us with endless information at the tap of a screen, the human lessons of nutrition, movement, and self-care are more vital than ever. It isn't a coincidence that there is a lot of news coverage of a youth mental health epidemic at the same time.

We cannot Google or large-language model the lived experience of resilience, balance, and physical well-being, the very skills that keep us from becoming another statistic in the sick care cycle. The actions young people take today will have a lasting impact on them later in life. The food they put in their mouths at age 17 will lay the foundation for their well-being at age 70. However, at age 17, there is simply no standard best practice in place to lay a foundation for choices made in the kitchen. At 70, it is too late to change course.

Research from the Harvard T.H. Chan School of Public Health shows that a plant-based diet can reduce the risk of heart disease by up to 25 percent and lower the odds of cognitive decline. Dean Ornish, MD, has long demonstrated how a combination of nutrition, movement and mindfulness can reverse the course of chronic disease. Contrary to popular belief, a 2023 JAMA analysis found that plant-based diets can be 25–29 percent less expensive when fewer animal products are included.

Sectionalization

When we cut school or health-access budgets, the most vulnerable always pay the price. This is the blind spot in policymaking: decisions framed as "savings" are often just deferred costs, kicked down a road already full of potholes. When the road crumbles, we all pay more to repair the damage.

Take Medicaid. Reasonable people can agree that those who are able to work should do so, both for their own dignity and for the benefit of taxpayers. But work requirements overlook a central reality: many adults cannot work consistently because childcare is unaffordable or unavailable. When more than ten million people lose Medicaid coverage, their health needs do not vanish. They still get sick, they still require care, and without coverage, they turn to emergency rooms, the most expensive and least efficient point of entry into the system. We tried this model in the 1980s and 1990s. It failed then. Yet, reliance on emergency rooms continues.

LBJ understood this truth when he championed Medicare and Medicaid, seeking to ensure that illness would not impoverish families. We reinforced that principle in 1986 with the Emergency Medical Treatment and Labor Act, which guaranteed that anyone arriving at an ER would receive care regardless of ability to pay. It was an important act of compassion. At the same time, it also created an unfunded mandate that left hospitals with enormous costs. When no single entity covers the cost, the burden ultimately falls on everyone through higher taxes and hospital costs.

Hospitals left to carry this burden inevitably face deficits. Hard choices follow: fewer nurses, delayed upgrades, or limits on care. None of those choices align with our shared purpose to heal.

The question is not whether people will need care; they will. The question is whether we build a system that meets those needs wisely and humanely, or one that waits until people are at the breaking point and then treats them in the most expensive and inefficient way possible. Empathy and foresight are not mere luxuries in health policy. They are common-sense tools that prevent today's cost-cutting from becoming tomorrow's crisis.

The government may have saved money, but in doing so, it has merely passed the hot potato to another sector of the health industry. The people who are sick are still sick. Hospitals will need to appeal to the state for subsidies. If subsidies are unavailable, hospitals will close their doors to those in need. We must face reality: sickness becomes the cost we all share, both economically and emotionally.

What happens if we have fewer hospitals and those struggling to stay open close their doors? In large cities, people will have to drive a few more minutes. In rural areas, people will have to drive several hours longer.

If state subsidies are an option, how will the subsidies be funded? Increased state taxes will fund the subsidies. The government may say, "Look, America. We've saved you billions." However, problems don't simply disappear. This is a deadly policy decision. It may save money at one level of government, but it will come at the expense of human lives. This is the inescapable result of fragmentation and short-term thinking.

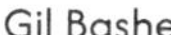

Perhaps the most powerful way to reduce sickness is to envision a system that prevents it. Yet, our financing model keeps the entire system on unstable ground. Most health professionals are still compensated through a fee-for-service model that rewards visits and volume, rather than prioritizing prevention or long-term health. A physician is reimbursed for the basics, such as reviewing diagnostics, checking blood tests, and reading X-rays, but not for the time it takes to keep a patient well.

To make a living as a physician, it's necessary to see many people quickly. We must collectively ask ourselves: how much time will a doctor have to sit down and educate a patient? For someone with a straightforward condition, a rushed visit may be frustrating but manageable. Yet, for people with complex or multi-system illnesses, patients juggling diabetes, heart disease, chronic pain, or mental health challenges, a short window of time can mean missed details, uncoordinated care, and worsening outcomes. The very patients who need more attention are often the ones least served by the system's pace.

Imagine if payers reimbursed patients for nutrition counseling or personal training? In addressing patient needs, it's more than defaulting to weight-loss drugs that treat obesity. Specialists are needed to address the too-often-overlooked cardiometabolic conditions. Yet, with some 100 trained obesity specialists in the United States, we need a system-wide approach.

Pioneers such as Louis J. Aronne, MD, FACP, the Sanford I. Weill Professor of Metabolic Research at Weill Cornell Medical Center, a leading authority on obesity and its treatment, are taking that uphill path. Dr. Aronne and his protégé, Katherine H. Saunders, MD, are seeking to make their expertise available nationwide, combining established science with entrepreneurism. Their challenge is to get the system to recognize that an ounce of prevention and earlier intervention is less costly than eventual sick care.

Keep People Alive to 65

In 1980, the average American could expect to live 73.7 years, a figure comparable to that of most other wealthy nations at the time. Yet, while life expectancy in Europe and Asia kept rising steadily, the U.S. began to stall. KFF Health News reports that decade by decade, the gap widened. Today, Americans not only spend more on healthcare than our global peers, but we also live shorter lives. How is this even possible?

The U.S. leads the world in medical talent, resources, and innovation. Our physicians, nurses, pharmacists, technicians, and administrators are among the highest-trained professionals globally. This makes sense, considering we spend nearly 18 percent of our GDP on health, some $4.5 trillion.

The U.S. has championed numerous recent scientific breakthroughs, including cancer therapies, life-saving cardiac devices, and AI-driven diagnostics. Despite this inventiveness, Americans live lives that are up to ten years shorter than those of people in other developed nations. In 2024, the Commonwealth Fund Mirror Report ranked the U.S. last among high-income nations in terms of access, equity, and health outcomes,

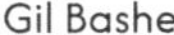

a disappointing grade for a system that spends more and delivers less than any peer country.

Millions of Americans still lack basic access to health services. This is a crisis of priorities, not scarcity. The U.S. health system isn't structured to prioritize improving people's health.

We don't need to spend more, dismantle the system, or wait for the perfect alignment of financial incentives to begin improving outcomes. Instead, we need to agree on a shared driver for decision-making, which should improve people's physical and mental well-being. Why not prioritize people's experience? Why not share a standard metric, such as patient outcomes?

When systems promote decisions that prioritize healthy lives, emergency visits decline, chronic conditions stabilize, and quality of life improves. This is not aspirational; it is proven. Recent evidence shows that coordinated care is not just a theory, but a proven intervention. A 2022 study in the American Journal of Managed Care found that structured patient-navigation programs reduced emergency department use by 32 percent among high-need patients, demonstrating the real power of proactive management to curb avoidable crises.

Aligning Profitability and Sustainability

The Federal government might tout the fact that budget reduction is saving money. However, these healthcare spending cuts transfer costs over to hospitals, which must appeal to the states. In turn, hospitals will have to appeal to their taxpayers. They can't merely print endless amounts of money. The reimbursing entity may change, but ultimately, the money still comes from taxpayers.

What do we do to prevent this? If you suddenly noticed your faucet was dripping, you could say, "That's bothering me. I'll put a cup under the drip and line it with a paper towel. Then, the water will fill the cup and flow into the drain. I won't hear the 'drip, drip, drip.'"

Is that actually a solution? Wouldn't it be more effective to say, "I'm going to call a plumber to fix it. That will not only get rid of the drip but also find the source and solve the problem." Unfortunately, today's sick care system only addresses the irritating noise of the drip, not the source of the leak.

As a modern and inventive society, how can we devise a better solution than quieting the drip? We need a system that recognizes when people are getting sick in "disease hotspots" and invests in addressing the root causes. A family of four still has to eat, even living on the poverty line, but might be eating Froot Loops and not fresh fruit?

What if food assistance programs like SNAP (the Supplemental Nutrition Assistance Program) or CHIP (the Children's Health Insurance Program) were designed not only to reduce hunger but also to make nutritious options easily accessible? The challenge is not just a lack of knowledge or a lack of desire. Families often understand what nutritious foods are, but affordability, availability, and time can get in the way. Ultimately, it is about creating conditions where food choices are not just known, but within people's reach, literally and figuratively.

When people become sick, the cost ripples across the entire system. Currently, Medicaid plays a key role in bailing out hospital systems, plugging holes rather than addressing the root causes of health inequities related to social determinants. Cutting one budget only to spend more elsewhere is not savings; it is a shell game that ultimately leaves the public paying more.

The reality is that economic hardship has a profound impact on health. Families with limited financial resources often reside in neighborhoods where healthy food is difficult to access; Federal data indicate that 18.8 million Americans live in areas officially classified as "low access," where affordable, nutritious options are scarce. Environmental risks follow similar lines. In a study published in 2014 in the International Journal of Hygiene and Environmental Health, children living near wood-processing factories faced a 74 percent higher risk of hospitalization for respiratory disease. This is a stark reminder that place, not just personal choice, shapes health long before a family reaches a clinic.

Yet, we rarely connect these dots in crafting the solutions. Budget debates often treat health costs, food access, and environmental conditions as separate issues when, in fact, they are deeply intertwined. Worse still, those who point out the ecological roots of illness are too often dismissed, as if these truths are an inconvenience rather than a lifeline. Empathy and collaboration are the human tools that reconnect these dots and remind us that health policy is people policy.

The current emphasis of policy is on economic development and prosperity. The economy's health is vital to the nation's well-being. We should also recognize that economics and health are intertwined. Preventive medicine is an investment that reaps rewards, financially and physically.

There is also the human aspect to consider. These are financial balance sheets and the ledger of humanity. They spill into each other. If humanity's balance sheet is off-kilter, it inevitably destabilizes the financial balance sheets of businesses and governments.

The dangers of neglect became clear to me early in my work in environmental health in the late 1980s. In Gadsden, Alabama, a smelting factory loomed over nearby homes. Its smoke was so corrosive that it ate the paint off houses every few years. The factory paid to repaint them, a cosmetic fix that maintained their appearance. However, if paint was peeling off wood, what was happening inside people's bodies? Covering the walls was cheaper than addressing the root cause with cleaner technology or medical care, but the real, human costs were still being paid.

This is what happens when we operate with a siloed mindset. Health, environment, education, and economics are treated like disconnected rooms in a building, each with locked doors. Decisions made in one room reverberate through the others, yet no one is walking the hallways to connect them. It may appear as a line-item savings on a corporate or government

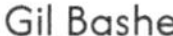

balance sheet, but the hidden deficit ultimately shows up on humanity's.

Solving problems like this requires breaking down those locked doors. How? By cultivating a collaborative spirit that treats people not as liabilities to be managed but as lives to be protected.

Instead, we're saddled with the sick care system and continue to sink money into it. The time has come to break the cycle. We must recognize the inescapable link between the environment and human health and find ways to harmonize these interests. We must return to eating healthier, more nutritious foods and raise children whose families can both find and afford them.

This approach requires effort at every level: policy, community, and family. Lawmakers, educators, and parents all need to understand how public health works in practice. Success lies in equipping each generation with the knowledge and support to have affordable choices and provide communities with the tools to act on them.

Small Interventions, Big Outcomes

One of the most compelling examples of this shift came from the work of Dr. Jeffrey Brenner, who catalyzed the formation of the Camden Coalition. Camden, New Jersey, across the river from Philadelphia, has long been one of the underinvested neighborhoods in the state. It is marked by high rates of illness, poverty, and violence, a place where despair and disease often seem to go hand in hand.

Dr. Brenner and his team examined patterns that others accepted as inevitable and posed different questions. The Camden Coalition gained widespread recognition for its "hotspotting" approach toward enhancing outcomes for individuals with chronic, unmanaged conditions. They asked an essential question: "Why were so many children coming into emergency rooms with severe asthma attacks?" The answer was not simply a matter of bad luck or genetics. Often, the genesis was environmental.

Treating the attacks was costly, but Dr. Brenner's team found it was far more effective to send a social worker into the home. In many cases, the solution was as practical as installing a $200 air conditioner to reduce triggers. That small intervention dramatically improved the quality of life and cut down repeat ER visits.

No doctor can prescribe an air conditioner, yet that simple tool did more to prevent illness than repeated hospitalizations. Brenner's insight was clear: health is shaped as much by environment as by medicine. His work showed that when we look beyond the walls of the clinic, we can find practical, humane, and cost-effective ways to reduce suffering.

As Dr. Brenner once shared in Kaiser Health News in 2011, "Emergency room visits and hospital admissions should be considered failures of the healthcare system until proven otherwise." That perspective reframes sickness not as a given but as a challenge to be prevented wherever possible. It also reminds us that sustainable enterprise in healthcare depends not only on innovation or revenue streams but on the ability to connect the dots between environment, community, policy, and patient needs.

Dr. Brenner's work reveals a simple yet profound truth: poverty and illness are inextricably linked. Where economic opportunity is absent, disease takes root. That reality is not confined to urban centers; it also extends into rural America.

In the Catskills, New York, once-vibrant towns by the mid-1990s had been hollowed out by economic decline, leaving residents with limited access to opportunity, culture, or even hope. Into that void stepped Peter and Sarah Finn, who understood that healing a community requires more than clinics or prescriptions; it requires dignity, creativity, and the belief that people deserve beauty and possibility in their daily lives.

Through the Catskill Mountain Foundation, the Finns reimagined the region as a place not of decline but of renewal. They invested in the arts, education, and economic development as levers of public health. Over the years, the Foundation has invested millions in facilities and programming, helping to anchor jobs and drive local economic growth in a historically fragile economy.

When people gather to learn, create, and connect, they strengthen both community fabric and economic resilience. What emerged was more than a cultural hub; it was a living demonstration that sustainability and health are intertwined. A community with access to opportunity is a community less vulnerable to despair and the cascade of illnesses born of poverty.

The Finns' work underscores a larger truth: sustainable health is not achieved solely through medicine. By fostering hope, education, and opportunity, they helped restore balance to a community that once seemed left behind. Their example reminds us that empathy and collaboration, applied to the roots of poverty, can transform not just individual lives but the destiny of entire communities.

Our ecosystem must adopt this collaborative, common-sense mindset if it is to fulfill its purpose. Preventive care, empathy, and structural awareness are not just moral imperatives; they are the most efficient path toward building an enduring health system that serves people.

The fragmented segments of the health system must rally together and declare, "We can sustain our businesses and still converge where it matters most. We can take a hotspot of disease and prove that collaboration shifts the illness trajectory." This is not an impossible dream; it is practical, measurable, and humane. When profit and purpose intersect, patients, professionals, and enterprises all benefit.

The health industry must generate profit to be sustainable, reinvest in science, and fuel innovation. Alongside these investments, we have the opportunity to shape a multi-layered payer system respected by society, not viewed as an adversary but as a partner in survival. We can create a system applauded for helping to secure a healthier future.

Just as cities require a master plan to connect neighborhoods and prevent sprawl, healthcare requires a guiding blueprint. Empathy and collaboration are that blueprint. They remind us that technology, science, and policy are tools, not ends in themselves. When we align those tools with purpose, when we measure success in both healthier lives and sustainable enterprise, we move from patching sickness to building wellness. With the right design, the system can thrive while truly serving the people it was built to heal.

Chapter 6

THE BLUEPRINT: COLLABORATION AND PATIENT-CENTERED CARE

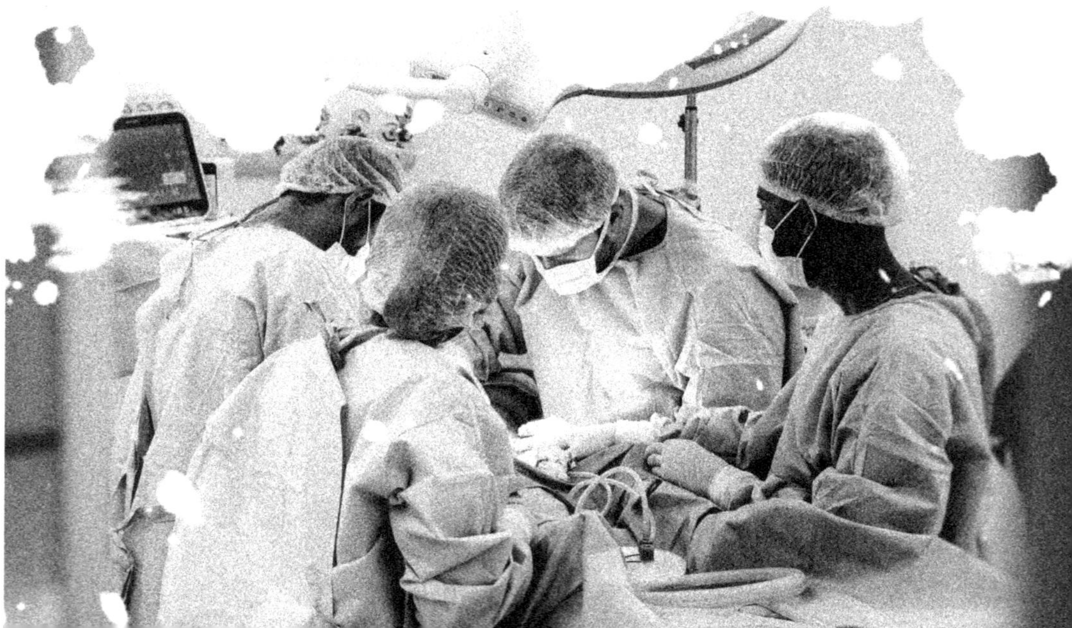

EVERY sector of the health industry answers to a different financial authority. Hospitals, payers, policymakers, biopharmaceutical companies, and device manufacturers all pursue their own incentives. What's missing is the one thing patients need most: collaboration. This absence is a public health crisis. Collaboration is not an inconvenience but the engine of better health outcomes.

The call for collaboration does not mean more technology, more software, or another round of industry "summits." It is not a cry for budget allocations or more continuing medical education. It is a call for something deeper: a recalibration of behaviors, mindsets, and values. Until we align around a shared purpose, the system will continue to serve itself instead of serving patients.

The cost of that misalignment is measured in lives. Health cannot be a contact sport. It is designed, when optimized, to be a team sport uniting the healer and the person seeking to be healed.

Health is a Team Sport

When my daughter first saw Dr. Nieca Goldberg at NYU Langone, what stood out was not only her clinical expertise but also her honesty. Dr. Goldberg had the courage to say, "I don't know." She added something equally vital, "You need a team." Her call-to-action captures the essence of collaboration. No single physician, no matter how skilled, can meet every need alone. It takes a team, coordinated, respectful, and human-centered, to surround patients with the care they deserve.

Collaboration between physicians and patients is at the heart of health and wellness. The data is clear: when health professionals are genuinely engaged, they look beyond symptoms to understand the patient's life journey. This engagement requires something simple yet scarce—time. When physicians have time to connect, trust grows. Trust, more than any test result, predicts whether patients follow guidance, return for care, and heal.

The best doctors I've met are both experts in their fields and remarkable in how they carry themselves. Their knowledge is unquestioned, yet what stands out is their humility. They listen with intensity and center their efforts around their patients' needs as part of the same care team.

Ultimately, we are not just cases or conditions. We are always people, and sometimes patients. A physician who clings to the illusion of being all-powerful is not a healer but a false idol. True medicine is built on skill, yes, but also on connection, respect, and humanity.

Doctors who remember that they are people and relate to patients as people tend to be better, dedicated health professionals. We can sense how much they care. This is key and automatically establishes a collaborative spark with their patients.

When doctors see the person before them, the relationship begins to take root. Yet our system reduces that human connection to Centers for Medicare and Medicaid Services (CMS) Star Rating or a patient survey response questionnaire. Grades sensitize people. We respect what we inspect, but it's not enough. Perhaps medical school admissions can heighten the emphasis on those who prioritize human connection alongside their MCAT scores.

The quality of the relationship between the care provider and the patient influences the patient's desire to engage with the health system and to listen to the direction or advice of health professionals. When we reduce patient time for the sake of efficiency, we remove the essential connection that enables strong patient relationships and better outcomes.

Part of the challenge is that the system itself lacks a shared metric by which all physicians and the ecosystem around them are evaluated. Today, reimbursement is primarily tied to procedures and volume rather than whether patients feel cared for or achieve better health outcomes. However, if physicians knew they were being evaluated based on their patients' experiences, the incentives would shift. Doctors would have reason not only to diagnose and treat but also to communicate clearly, listen carefully, and build trust. The result would be a system that rewards healing relationships, not just transactions, and that produces both better experiences and better outcomes.

CMS considers consumer reaction a viable metric. If long-term care facility residents are unhappy, that facility is likely to see few inbound referrals. Quality and experience can impact the topline. Yet think about people with dementia. The sickest among us often cannot speak up, and that is precisely why empathy cannot be optional and must be built into every corner of the system. Leaders have a responsibility to act with urgency, balancing two key priorities: protecting the patient experience and confronting the rising costs of care. This is not a delicate balance to admire; it is a mandate to meet.

We must make the patient experience and patient satisfaction scoring transparent. Instead of saying, "We're the best in this category," health entities should say, "Our patient experience is the best. Here's the score, and here's why."

CMS also ranks hospitals based on patient experience. One key measure is the "patient survey rating," which reflects how patients felt during their hospital stay. Recently discharged patients were asked about essentials that shape trust in care: how clearly doctors and nurses communicated, how responsive staff were to their needs, and even the basics of cleanliness and quiet. These details may seem small, but together they reveal whether a hospital truly delivers a healing environment.

Hospitals nationwide care for millions of Medicare and Medicaid beneficiaries each year. Most hospitals that participate in Medicare and have sufficient data carry CMS Star Ratings, a public scorecard found on the Medicare Care Compare website, that includes patient-experience measures. These ratings are easy to overlook, yet they tell a consistent story about how people feel inside the system.

Unlike glossy marketing claims, CMS patient-experience scores are public disclosures. If a hospital proclaims, "We have the nation's best oncologists," its patient-experience rating should stand beside that claim. Transparency is not a luxury; it is the foundation of trust. A hospital may invest in cutting-edge technology, yet if patients report poor communication, long waits, or indifference, those realities should carry as much weight as awards for clinical excellence.

The distinction is critical. U.S. News & World Report, Newsweek, and Time highlight centers of excellence in oncology, cardiology, and orthopedics. CMS rankings measure something entirely different: whether patients felt heard and respected. Clinical skills and innovation save lives. However, empathy determines whether people trust the health system, return for follow-up care, and recommend it to others.

When hospitals invest in communication and patient understanding, the results are measurable. A 2021 JAMA Network meta-analysis found that enhanced discharge communication reduced 30-day readmissions from 13.5 to 9.1 percent, a roughly one-third reduction, while also improving adherence and patient satisfaction. In the end, excellence in medicine cannot exist without excellence in empathy.

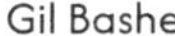

Collaboration

That same misalignment plays out beyond the bedside. It surfaces in every administrative battle between doctors and payers, where the focus is on cost containment rather than on people's lived experiences. Collaboration grounded in empathy, not just efficiency, must guide both clinical and administrative decisions if the system is to earn trust.

When doctors seek prior authorization for tests and treatments, the request is reviewed against payer policies. The stated purpose is appropriateness and cost control. Friction arises when those policies diverge from clinical judgment or miss the patient's context. The first line of review is often conducted by non-clinical administrative staff following scripted criteria, with escalations to nurses and, ultimately, a medical director when needed. That structure can leave the treating clinician feeling that a patient's needs are being judged at a distance, through rules rather than relationship.

Transparent payer-experience metrics would help. Imagine a public scorecard that reports prior-authorization turnaround times, initial denial rates, appeal overturn rates, and clarity of communication. Plans would compete on ease and equity, not just price. Research also shows that patient-experience scores can vary by type of insurance coverage, not only by the care delivered. This penalizes clinicians for factors beyond their control. In plain terms, a patient's insurance benefits can skew how their care is judged. This is yet another reason to adjust how performance is measured so that payers, providers, and patients are finally pulling in the same direction.

In a fee-for-service world, a specialist earns a living by doing the work a patient needs. One gate stands between clinical judgment and care: prior authorization. A health plan can approve or deny. Without approval, there is no procedure, no payment, and often no relief. Who holds the power? Not the physician at the bedside or the patient in pain, but the entity controlling the checkbook, far from the exam room.

Payers are designed to act as actuaries of care, pricing risk, enforcing coverage policies, and adjudicating claims. That mindset shows up in how they label us: beneficiaries, not customers. We depend on coverage to avoid financial ruin; without it, bankruptcy is a real risk. The irony is obvious: without people to cover, payers have no business. We are not supplicants; we are the market.

I have felt the asymmetry. Even after contributing significantly to premiums and unreimbursed out-of-pocket costs (with my employer also paying), I am treated less like a customer and more like an item on an assembly line to be scanned. If plans can veto care, then accountability must meet authority: measure how quickly they say yes, how fairly they say no, and how clearly they explain the path to "approved."

I confront the system; my physician confronts it with me. The payer makes the call. That gatekeeper has little incentive to smooth the path. The result is a tension that should not exist, yet it defines the entire healthcare experience for millions.

Guardrails are reasonable. Coverage decisions must protect appropriateness and control waste. There is a line, however. When a plan denies treatment to a paying member, the consequence is not mere bureaucracy.

For some, it can become a medical cliff—the difference between stability and spiraling decline, sometimes life and death. For example, cancer patients who face weeks of prior authorization delays for chemotherapy know that every lost day gives the disease more ground. That moment is the tipping point to despair. Patients know it. Clinicians know it. Payers know it too.

Still, the machine grinds on. Members continue to pay premiums and deductibles, only to have their expected care refused—tests, therapies, and procedures they thought would be covered. In those moments, the balance sheet benefits while families absorb the human cost in fear, delays, and deteriorating health.

Each part of the system is driven by a fundamentally different economic parameter. Unlike the clothing business, where the buyer knows the exact costs throughout the supply chain, the healthcare system is far more complex. Each entity generates revenue in a unique manner, and one entity may not fully understand how another entity generates its income.

The public often believes our health system works as a single, holistic community. In reality, it functions like an archipelago, with islands of care connected by fragile bridges. Each island optimizes for its own incentives, so patients do the island-hopping, paperwork in hand.

That fragmentation shows up in how we pay for care. Prior authorization and fee schedules judge individual procedures, not whole-person needs. Even when a clinician advocates for a broader plan, reimbursement typically reverts to the code: pay for this test and that surgery. However, anything beyond the narrow indication falls outside the scope.

Research bears this out: individuals with higher BMI are several times more likely to experience rotator cuff tears or require surgical repair, with one case-control study showing that people with a BMI of 35 or greater were three times more likely to undergo shoulder repair than those of normal weight (CDC-supported study, Bailey et al., 2023). These are not abstract statistics; they are design cues for how we should structure care and payment.

A collaborative approach would look beyond the operating room and ask, "What prevents the other shoulder or the repair itself from failing?" Payers and providers could contract for the full episode of care, addressing not only the surgery but also its drivers, including nutrition support, supervised activity, behavioral coaching, and follow-up that helps patients maintain weight loss and best manage pain. Prevention is part of the outcome.

The fix is straightforward: pay for results across the whole episode, not just the incision. Tie reimbursement to fewer avoidable revisions, better function, and sustained weight improvement. When payers and clinicians share those metrics, the islands connect, and patients experience a system that finally works as one.

What happens if payers say, "Your patient needs a knee replacement? You got it. What's the game plan to help the patient lose weight so we don't have to replace the other knee, which is very expensive?" Establishing a common plan for these very scenarios would be both collaborative and profitable. When the system begins to acknowledge cause and effect and chooses to actively work to prevent adverse outcomes, money will be saved, profits will increase, and lives will be enhanced.

Too often, we treat the cost of a second surgery as unavoidable when the real opportunity is to invest in prevention across the entire episode of care, reducing avoidable revisions and improving long-term outcomes. Payers genuinely try to help by assigning care navigators to guide patients through the system. However, those navigators often narrow, rather than broaden, the path, steering patients toward in-network, lower-cost options that may not fully meet their needs.

All of this is complex. Shoulder problems are not always directly tied to BMI, despite research often assuming this connection. When a person is in pain and can't lift or move their arm, exercise becomes difficult. This is the classic chicken-and-egg dilemma. What matters most is not assigning blame, but ensuring patients feel heard. A physician who listens, engages with the person rather than just the body part, and understands the full context of their life can make all the difference.

See the Whole Person

Empathy isn't a soft skill; it is a clinical tool that improves outcomes and humanizes healthcare. Physician-author Dr. Jerome Groopman posits in his 2006 The New Yorker article that data does not replace presence. Statistics cannot substitute for the human being before you; statistics embody averages, not individuals. Every patient has a unique backstory, a path that leads them to the clinic door. When physicians learn about a patient's journey along that path, they gain context and insight.

These systemic blind spots show up even in something as simple as a "customer" letter. A single letter can decide whether care moves forward. Too many read like gibberish—dense legalese that obscures basic next steps. This is fixable. Plain language can turn a denial or "missing info" notice into actionable guidance that treats people with respect.

Recently, our plan mailed me a notice addressed to the "provider." It said reimbursement information was incomplete and demanded "our code." I am not a physician. I work in health policy and communications, and I am the plan's customer. That letter should have gone to my physician, with a clear copy to me explaining what was needed and by when. Instead, the system shifted the administrative burden to the patient, accidentally or not. In that moment, I was not a customer. I was invisible.

Almost unbelievably, my daughter received an insurance letter demanding that she explain why a neurologist had monitored her surgery, a procedure completed more than a year earlier, and to submit medical records, lab results, and operative reports she had no access to. How can a patient be expected to complete a task that even seasoned health professionals struggle to interpret?

If payers have the power to pause care, they also have the responsibility to communicate clearly. Every notice should state—in the first three lines—what is missing, who is responsible for sending it, the deadline, a live phone number, or a helpful online contact and appeal rights. Route clinical requests to clinicians; send patients a plain-English summary of status and next steps. That is not marketing. That is care.

This is where communication itself becomes part of care. A simple review could have stopped that letter. Someone might have asked, "Will this confuse or frighten the patient? Shouldn't their physician be the one to explain?" Yet no one asked. That silence speaks volumes. In a system that claims to serve patients, the most basic questions of empathy and clarity are too often forgotten.

Some physicians make empathy part of the protocol, not performance. Dr. Rafael Grossmann, a trauma and general surgeon based in Portsmouth, New Hampshire, is one of them. He is willing to forgo an operation when an equally effective, safer path exists. His reputation rests not only on technical excellence, but also on judgment—the wisdom to know that the best procedure is sometimes no procedure at all.

In consultations, Dr. Grossmann begins with the person's goals, not their list of problems. His first question is simple yet transformative, "What are you hoping to get back to?" If a nonoperative plan can help a patient reach that goal, that is the path he recommends.

He pulls his chair level with the patient, translates complex options into plain language, and writes out clear next steps they can follow at home. Learners may see him using mixed-reality tools to teach surgery from the clinician's vantage point, but what patients remember most is that he looked them in the eye and stayed present through their fear. His invitation, "Don't call me doctor, call me Rafael," softens the hierarchy and opens the conversation. When that wall drops, better information comes to the surface. Better choices follow.

When policy gets in the way of good care, he advocates for change. He gathers evidence, escalates appropriately, and makes the case for what the patient needs. That persistence isn't theater—it's care. Skill matters. Presence matters. And so does the willingness to challenge a system that gets in the way of healing.

Training more physicians like Dr. Grossmann must begin long before the operating room. Admissions should value curiosity and listening alongside test scores. Training programs must assess how clearly clinicians communicate under pressure—not just how precisely they operate. Mentorship should reward habits such as clear explanations, shared decisions, and the humility to avoid unnecessary procedures, so that technical mastery becomes synonymous with human healing.

Product innovators already understand this principle. Real-world success depends on the people being served. They bring patients into every stage of development and marketing, listening closely to what works in practice. The same should apply across healthcare. For hospitals, that means recognizing that every outcome is shaped not just by treatment or surgery, but by how patients feel about their care. For payers, it means acknowledging that communication and decision-making affect more than budgets—they shape people's well-being and, often, their medical outcomes.

Getting this right doesn't require dismantling the system. It requires measuring success differently. Every organization must track costs, revenue, and sustainability—but they must also prioritize experience, satisfaction, and the human story. If a patient says, "I got what I needed, but you made my life miserable," then the system has failed, regardless of how good the clinical outcome appears on paper.

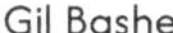

No transformation is possible unless the system holds itself accountable for patient experience. Respect begins with respect for a person's data, their voice, and their dignity. When those elements are honored, innovation and policy can finally deliver on their promise.

Systems rarely reform themselves. It's patients and families who push them to change.

The Power of the Patient Voice

Even the most empathetic physician cannot shift the system alone. Patient advocacy transforms individual pain into organized change. It isn't a side channel; it's a force that keeps institutions honest and aligned with human outcomes. People deserve to be heard. When they are not, frustration hardens into distrust. Advocacy converts that frustration into organizing, evidence, and progress.

Advocacy takes many forms, including national organizations, local nonprofits, online communities, and the steady persistence of individuals. Each plays a vital role. Formal groups give patients a collective identity and a seat at the table. Experienced patients help newcomers interpret diagnoses and navigate treatment options. Online forums can serve as lifelines of knowledge and solidarity, even with their imperfections. Survivorship bias and self-selection can tilt conversations toward those still struggling, but when used thoughtfully, these communities reveal barriers, share workarounds, and spread information faster than any brochure.

Real-world evidence strengthens that collective voice. Platforms like StuffThatWorks, founded by Yael Elish, allow patients to document their journeys, track outcomes, and compare what truly helps in everyday life. This kind of evidence doesn't replace clinical trials; it complements them. It adds context that trials can't always capture. This may include side effects that affect daily routines, access barriers that hinder adherence, and patterns suggesting more effective therapy sequencing. This is patient voice transformed into actionable insight—evidence that clinicians, payers, and policymakers can use to make better decisions.

Yet, because this data frequently falls outside traditional clinical protocols, it's often dismissed as "unverified" or "not FDA-recognized." Such dismissal overlooks a profound truth: there is immense value in listening to lived experience. Patients' firsthand accounts reveal how the healthcare system truly functions—or fails—in real life.

While this real-world data is gathered outside controlled environments, it offers a panoramic view of medicine as experienced by those living it. From medication access to symptom management, these insights shed light on realities that official sources often struggle to capture. They allow us to see illness through the patient's eyes—to walk, however briefly, in their shoes. That perspective is indispensable.

Until the industry accepts the patient's voice as valid evidence—not as anecdote but as essential data—patients will remain outside the conversation. How can satisfaction matter if the voice behind it doesn't count? A person's experience is their reality. When many people report similar experiences, those stories form a signal, not noise.

Other sectors learned this lesson long ago. Retailers and airlines monitor social channels in real time, respond to complaints, and adjust operations because customer input predicts performance. A clothing brand that hears, "Great sport coats, weak tie selection," heeds the voice of its customers. A premier airline passenger who reports a delay is contacted by a trained service team empowered to resolve the issue and follow through. These industries treat feedback as operational data—a leading indicator of revenue and loyalty—not as public relations material or a box to check.

That's the micro-level insight in aggregate—critical data too often ignored.

There is no shortage of examples showing positive health outcomes driven by real-world advocacy. The AIDS movement of the 1980s and 1990s is one of the most powerful. When patient activists and HIV-positive individuals rallied together, they forced the biopharma industry, hospital systems, and the government to prioritize HIV-related treatments. Their determination saved countless lives.

Patient advocacy does more than raise awareness; it changes trajectories. Consider Let's Win Pancreatic Cancer, a collaboration between advocates and clinicians. The platform crowdsources clinical trials, real-world experiences, and practical guidance. The result is earlier trial matching, faster access to treatment options, and a tangible sense of direction for families facing a fast-moving disease. The model is simple yet powerful, putting knowledge in the hands of patients and the clinicians who support them.

The same dynamic applies to less-publicized conditions. Arrhythmia advocacy groups, for example, have elevated irregular heartbeats from private concern to public health priority. They educate primary care teams, shape screening and referral pathways, and press for policies that improve access to diagnostics and therapies. Different diseases, same lesson: organized patients, working alongside engaged clinicians, move systems.

The implication is immediate. If lived experience is evidence, then advocacy is the engine that turns it into action. Health systems should invite advocacy groups to co-design educational materials, integrate trial navigation into clinic workflows, and use patient-reported data to address friction points. That is how the "patient experience" becomes part of care delivery itself, not just a rating after the fact.

Clinical culture matters too. We need more physicians who treat surgery as a last resort and fewer who dismiss patient reports with lines like, "Who are you going to believe, a patient or me?" That reflex captures the larger problem. The antidote is partnership—listen first, align on outcomes, and choose the least invasive plan that helps a person return to their life.

If the patient voice is still missing, it is because each part of the system is busy optimizing for its own needs. Hospitals must stay solvent, payers manage risk, and clinicians manage time. Patients, however, need a life they recognize. When advocates unite with supportive physicians and health professionals, priorities shift—coverage decisions become clearer, navigation simpler, and satisfaction rises because care finally reflects what people value. That is not hype or idealism; it is how the system is designed to serve the patient, rather than by accident.

A powerful example is The Marfan Foundation, an advocacy community that champions research and patient support for connective tissue disorders, reminding us of the importance of early diagnosis and coordinated care in improving quality of life and longevity. I am honored to serve on the advocacy board of this game-changing group. This nonprofit has earned exceptional ratings for transparency and impact, including a top score from Charity Navigator. The services it provides for patients with Marfan syndrome are extraordinary.

Each year, The Marfan Foundation convenes patients and families at a major medical center—not for another lecture, but for connection and care. People living with Marfan syndrome sit face-to-face with leading specialists, often for the first time, and receive consultations at no cost. Teens find strength in peer support groups where they can share their thoughts and feelings. Parents, carrying years of worry, gather in circles to compare notes, share hope, and discover they are not alone. Support groups continue throughout the year as well.

At the same time, the Foundation channels funding into research that pushes science forward. For too long, Marfan syndrome has been relegated to the margins of medicine. These gatherings show what happens when advocacy transforms an underserved condition into a community and then into a movement.

When patients find each other, scattered stories become signals, and those signals grow into critical mass. Voice turns into data. Data hardens into science. Science fuels communication that moves policy and practice. This is the pattern: connection leads to evidence, which leads to action.

This is how rare-disease communities become visible. They build registries, map symptoms, compare outcomes, and share what works. Fundraising follows, then studies and clinical trials. Clinicians start to listen, payers begin to adjust, and families feel less isolated.

Belonging is not sentiment. It is care. Inclusion is not a slogan. It is infrastructure.

Outcomes Over Office Visits

We must share a common goal if we are to create meaningful change in healthcare—a focus on patient experience and outcomes. The system must exist for its ultimate customer: the patient.

Currently, it appears that the healthcare system exists primarily for itself, rather than for the people it is intended to serve. That truth is uncomfortable but undeniable. Ask a simple question: Who is the customer? For payers, it is the payer. For providers, it is institutional viability. For policymakers, compliance with regulations is essential. Each part of the system orbits its own interests, protects its own budgets, and chases its own goals. The result is a self-serving system while patients wait at the margins, unseen. Until the system reclaims the patient as its true customer, no amount of money, policy, or innovation will bring the change we need.

No one is saying, "We commit to the common good of this one audience, and this is how we will impact them. We do not want people to enter the world sick. We want to prevent illness and provide care. If they fall ill, we want to help them recover. If they have chronic disease, we want to minimize its severity. We want them to feel that their lives matter."

That is not what the system is doing right now.

Physicians, especially primary care doctors in private practice, struggle to earn a living while covering rising costs for insurance, office space, and staff. Hospitals are trying to stay open. Policymakers are focused on enforcing regulations that contain the Federal budget.

No one in power is asking the most basic questions: What happens when people get sick? Who will care for them? Who will pay for that care? Policymakers debate trimming budgets but rarely discuss protecting lives. The silence is deafening. Instead of planning for people, the system plans for itself, because today, the system's customer is itself. Until that changes, patients will continue to be an afterthought.

Collaboration becomes possible when there is a shared metric, goal, and vision. The system does not currently operate in that manner. Every part of it operates for its own benefit. As long as this myopic approach to medicine continues, no substantial change will occur. The solution is within reach; it requires only mindful behavior.

A teacher, a parent, and a child share a metric: they want to feel happy, fulfilled, and successful, knowing that the child's needs, talents, and future are prioritized and nurtured. The parent does not say, "I'm so happy my kid is miserable but smart. The teacher is doing a good job toughening them up for the future." That is not the goal.

Parents listen to whether their children are excited about learning. Teachers feel fulfilled when students are enthusiastic about applying new knowledge. Children who enjoy learning earn higher test scores. The shared outcome centers on the child becoming a lifelong learner.

What is the shared metric in the health system? For payers, it is the adjudication of care. As physician practices consolidate into larger groups and hospitals merge, the long-standing relationships that once defined care are rarely preserved. A surgeon may see a patient three or four times. A gastroenterologist might see someone once or twice every five years for a colonoscopy. So, what is the shared metric? A repaired hernia? Removed polyps?

Augmented Implementation

Dr. Rafael Grossmann utilizes advanced technology—similar to virtual reality glasses—to provide students with a first-person view of the surgical procedure. While he operates in the OR, his students can observe from the gallery, seeing each step through his eyes as if standing beside him.

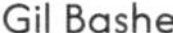

Dr. Grossmann has seen, time and again, that outcomes are shaped not only by what happens in the operating room but by the entirety of the patient's journey. A flawlessly executed cancer surgery cannot always overcome the biology of disease. What endures most is not just surgical technique, but the relationship. Patients recall how Dr. Grossmann listened, treated them with respect, and made them feel less alone. They remember the surgeon who cared for them as a person, not merely as a procedure.

When I interviewed him, he shared a blunt truth: in the age of artificial intelligence, information is instant. Yet, medical training still devotes years to memorizing physiology, chemistry, and biology—foundations that matter deeply. The opportunity now is to rebalance. Teach clinicians to use technology effectively in the operating room. Train clinical judgment. Prioritize curiosity, empathy, and an inquisitive approach to patient relationships. The next great medical skill is not recall—it is discernment, translation, and presence.

Knowledge alone does not heal. What matters is how that knowledge is used in the service of people. When clinical expertise is paired with mindfulness and compassion, outcomes shift. Patients feel seen, heard, and cared for—not processed. That is where science meets humanity.

This is why the debate around medical technology matters. Innovation is vital; technology can diagnose earlier, track patterns, and extend the reach of care. However, it cannot replace the human connection that makes healing possible. Machines can analyze, but only people can comfort, make meaning, and restore dignity. Technology will continue to advance, and clinicians will integrate new tools into their cognitive and physical skill sets. Yet, humanity, not hardware, must remain the organizing principle of care.

It is the human touch that transforms treatment into healing. As patients, our experiences with healthcare professionals can leave us feeling confident, cared for, listened to, and connected to the healing process. Our fascination with technology should never overshadow the millennia-old understanding that caring presence is the ultimate healer.

As John Whyte, MD, CEO of the American Medical Association, reminds us in a 2025 LinkedIn post, "... physicians must remain at the center of care. As AI grows in influence, it is critical that clinicians lead its design, implementation, and governance, not only to ensure its effectiveness but to safeguard the values that define our profession."

Accountable Care Organizations (ACOs) were established to transition us away from fragmented, reactive treatment and toward coordinated, value-based care. They are building a model that aligns outcomes with costs; margin-aware: not built to maximize profit. If they cannot stay solvent, they cannot fulfill their role of aligning care with value. The lesson is simple: without margin, mission cannot survive and without mission, margin has no purpose.

Kaiser Permanente, Advocate Health Care, and UCSF Health are strong examples of Accountable Care Organizations (ACOs) that demonstrate what is possible when collaboration and mission are aligned. They represent sustainable models that others can learn from and emulate. Excellence is not confined to any single structure.

Extraordinary performance is not a corporate form; it is a discipline. Publicly traded systems, community hospitals, and independent networks can all achieve it. The constant across models is simple: money must follow mission. Organizations that prioritize people, whether private, public, or nonprofit, earn trust, foster connections, and sustain their success.

When I ask business leaders, “What is your goal? What is your mission?” I often hear, “Grow from $2.0 to $2.6 billion in 18 months.” Growth may fund care, but it is not the North Star. A person facing a life-and-death decision is not comforted by a revenue target. They want to know: Will you see me, treat me well, and help me get my life back on track?

Profit is a legitimate goal for a hospital system—not as the mission, but as its fuel. Margin enables mission: hiring great clinicians, acquiring modern equipment, maintaining safe facilities, and continually answering the baseline question, “Why do we exist?”

That framing defines the ACO model. Within ACOs, clinicians, hospitals, and health professionals coordinate care around one guiding question: How do we work together for the good of the patient? It is more than an economic structure; it is a mindset.

When that question guides decisions, organizations can become focused and efficient. Resources, data, and expertise align toward one outcome: better health and better experience. Metrics shift from siloed profit and throughput to shared measures of healing. This is why patient satisfaction reliably rises in these models; the system is organized around the person.

The same principle should guide the wider ecosystem. Biopharma and device innovators succeed not only when they earn revenue or regulatory approval but when their therapies improve lives in the real world. Policymakers should design incentives that reward connection and coordination rather than fragmentation and delay. When profit is measured by the same yardstick as outcomes, the entire system—from payers to providers, innovators to regulators—begins to serve one mission.

This is the inflection point: when a health ecosystem chooses patient outcomes as its North Star, efficiency and profit emerge as consequences, not commands. Purpose drives performance. Alignment converts cost into value. Connection builds trust, making every plan more possible.

We must measure success by restoring lives, removing friction, and returning time to families. Trust is the currency of care and the balance sheet that compounds across generations. The engine of that trust is empathy—the one resource no system should function without.

Chapter 7

EMPATHY: REDEFINING THE SECTOR'S PURPOSE

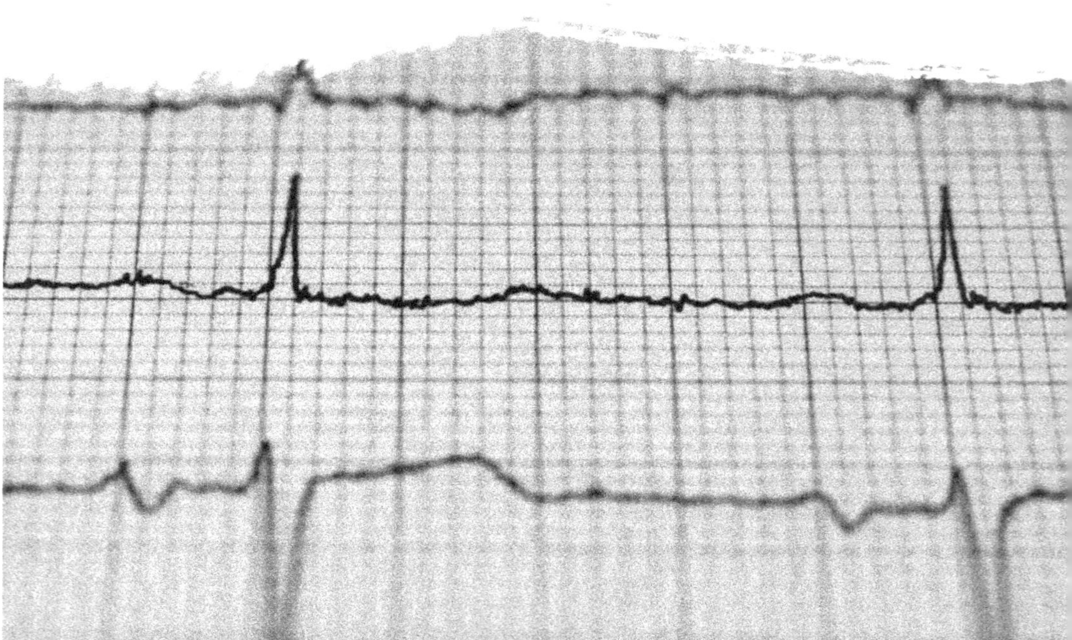

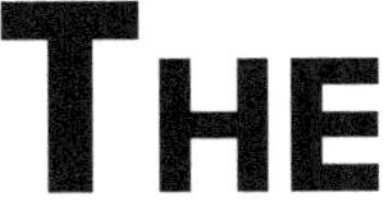

primary function of any health system is to support people's health. It sounds simple, and it should be.

Technology, innovation, finance, infrastructure, climate control, and transportation are all essential parts of the system, yet they exist for one reason only: to serve people. Without empathy at the center, these tools risk becoming ends in themselves rather than means to better care.

Empathy is the foundation that holds the system accountable to its purpose. A health system that encourages, nurtures, educates, and elevates empathy and embeds it into its culture will always be closer to achieving its true mission: serving humanity.

Too often, our healthcare delivery system is hindered by financially driven micro-priorities that obstruct efforts to improve people's well-being. Payers, product innovators, regulators, legislators, and policymakers each play vital roles, yet their competing models dominate the conversation so completely that caring for people is pushed to the margins. Their influence has grown so large that the broader voice of humanity, the very reason the system exists, is filtered out of the decision-making process.

In this environment, empathy risks becoming a metric, something to be tallied like inventory. However, health is not uniform or interchangeable. It is profoundly personal. What one person requires to stay well or recover may be entirely different from what another needs. This is why every advancement, policy, and innovation must return to a central question: Does this strengthen our bond to the people we serve?

I saw the importance of this question vividly when I visited a friend with stage IV cancer. I entered his hospital room as both a clergy member and a friend, but also as someone deeply familiar with the health system, with a background in business, communications, and medicine.

Prioritizing emotional and physical care made me attentive to details that others might overlook—from the room's condition and the staff's attentiveness to the range of therapies available, and even the writing on the whiteboard. Was it filled in? If so, what guidance did it signal to floor staff and family? Every signal revealed something about whether the system was truly serving him as a person, not just as a patient.

Yet beyond systems and checklists, I was there as a friend, mindful of his wife's burden, their daughter's worry, and the joy and hope a new grandchild brought into their lives. In those moments, simple questions mattered: How are you holding up? How is your daughter? Tell me about your granddaughter.

I was also present as clergy, concerned for their spiritual and emotional well-being. His wife and I spoke quietly about what the doctors had said, and I tried to bring clarity to a conversation that had left her overwhelmed. My goal was to interpret the medical facts and help her see the human dimensions behind them.

"The doctor looks at your husband through a clinical lens," I explained. "He has this cancer, at this stage, and the best practice is this treatment. His judgment is sound, and the protocols are appropriate."

"But medicine is not only about protocols," I continued. "It helps to ask, what facts did the doctor use to reach this decision? Which variables are driving the plan? Understanding that will give you confidence in the reasoning." She nodded, reassured that the medical judgment was accurate.

Then I shifted the frame. "There is another dimension, the human one. Medicine treats the body, but healing must also touch the soul. You have a new granddaughter. What will give your husband the most meaningful, comfortable time possible? What will make these days feel whole?"

That question shifted the conversation. She repeated again and again, "That is very helpful," because she understood what often gets lost in the fire of treatment: fighting for life is not only about time gained, but also about presence sustained.

When I visit people as a clergy member and the family leaves the room, I often have a very frank conversation with the person lying in a hospital bed. Beyond the stiff upper lip and instinctual competitiveness of fighting for your life, I ask them, “How are you really doing?”

Sometimes, they will tell me, “I’m so tired of this.” When they say that, I respond by asking, “What would you like to do? What would you like to see happen?”

Not infrequently, when a person is tired, they will say, “I’d like to be comfortable. I just want to go home.” In these cases, they will have been supportive of their family’s desire to fight the cancer, and although they’re now exhausted, they will be reluctant to admit to their family that maybe they’ve done all they can. They’ve done their best, but now all they want is to be comfortable.

I learned a lot from my father-in-law. He was well-versed in microbes and viruses, and he was an expert in diagnosing and treating liver disease, with a particular emphasis on hepatitis. He was the lead author of several major papers on hepatitis. Later, he returned to medical school and became a psychiatrist. His love for track and field led him to focus on the psychological well-being of athletes.

Of the final 13 days of his life, 12 were spent in a hospital. The medical protocols in place would have kept him there on the 13th day. My wife is a psychologist and has many patients who suffer from chronic illness. In many ways, she was his professional protégé.

My 97-year-old father-in-law had already voiced his desire to go home. He said, “No more hospitals.” We all knew what that meant. He wanted to pass in his own bed at home.

My wife pointedly asked the doctor, “Why are you keeping him here?”

The doctor said, “We’re keeping him here until we get hospice set up at the house.”

She clarified, “So, he doesn’t need to be here?”

The doctor said, “No.”

She said, “Well, in that case, I’d like my father to go home tonight rather than stay for our convenience.”

When the stretcher entered the house, my wife said, “Dad, you’re home.”

He said, “Yippie,” and gave a thumbs up!

On the night before Dr. Burt Giges drew his final breath, after a long, illustrious career and remarkable life, he was brought home. Less than 24 hours later, he closed his eyes, content in the one place on this planet where he would be most comfortable.

Empathy is not merely about being kind. It is about asking deeper questions: Am I doing this for you or for me? Am I supporting the patient, the doctor, the nurse, the pharmacist, and the technician in ways that matter? What am I doing to support you from a position of caring and understanding? Have we both made meaningful contributions to the reality of a shared outcome?

How do our communication, engagement, policies, and economic pathways impact the very people we are charged with serving? Who is the person at the corporate or government level responsible for asking, “Do these policies, or does this language, connect us to the very people we seek to serve? Or is it another wall we’re putting up that will inevitably stoke hostility?”

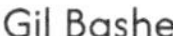

Joseph Heller's 1961 book Catch-22, about World War II bomber pilots, reflects the unhealthy paradox that has taken root in modern healthcare. A combat pilot will be deemed "unfit for battle" if they are willing to continue flying in deadly missions. However, if a combat pilot asks to be relieved of duty because they are "unfit for battle," it demonstrates a mind sane enough to be concerned with self-preservation, which would mean they are rational enough to continue bombing missions.

Ronald David (R.D.) Laing, MD, the Scottish psychiatrist who penned the compelling book The Divided Self: An Existential Study in Sanity and Madness, put it more plainly. He argued in 1960 that what we call schizophrenia may sometimes be a sane response to an insane world. Similarly, the anger and exhaustion of patients, physicians, nurses, payers, and policymakers alike can be viewed as rational responses to a system that has strayed far from its original mission.

The mission has never changed: to prevent illness and support health. Everything else, infrastructure, innovation, economics, and engagement, exists to serve that goal. The questions should be simple: Am I advancing prevention? Am I advancing healing? Am I investing in wellness? Am I creating pathways that return people from sickness to health? Am I making care more accessible, more hospitable, more humane?

What about the caregivers themselves? How can we expect empathy to flow if those providing care are treated without empathy? If the hours are relentless, if visits are rushed, if there is no room for pride in one's craft, how can we expect professionals to give their best to those who rely on them? To restore purpose, we must restore dignity for both patients and providers.

Imagine a mechanic who grew up helping his dad in the garage. He can replace a set of brakes in less than an hour and gets a job replacing brakes at a local repair shop. His new boss tells him that once he gets the car on the lift in the bay, he has to replace the brakes in only half an hour. How long will it be before a shoddy brake job costs lives?

When time is only measured in money, emotional outcomes become irrelevant. We are living in a world of conveyor-belt medicine. It brings to mind Charlie Chaplin caught in the grinding gears of Modern Times, or Lucille Ball frantically trying to keep up with chocolates spilling down the conveyor belt. In both scenes, the human being is overwhelmed by the very system meant to make life easier. Efficiency takes a human toll. In healthcare, innovation can fall into the same trap.

A new device powered by artificial intelligence should free clinicians to spend more time with patients, strengthening the human connection. Too often, however, the time saved is directed toward seeing more patients rather than being fully present with the ones already in the room. Our health system is designed to get more brakes replaced more quickly, not to make drivers safer.

With empathy as the guiding principle, all the technology, innovation, economics, and infrastructure center around our humanity. Empathy is the strategic driver that makes the system's pieces work better. It is not a matter of physicians engaging in small talk to be nicer; it is about true collaboration to forge partnerships.

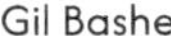

Unfortunately, we have flipped the process of care delivery. Increasingly, money is taking the lead over people's care outcomes. This is the heart of the issue.

We have to look at basic metrics collectively. Are we reducing non-communicable diseases? Are we, as a system, reducing the severity of heart disease, prediabetes, high cholesterol, heart attack, and stroke? Are we investing in strategies that prevent disease?

We have to look at patient satisfaction scores in terms of awareness and education. How does the patient feel about the treatment experience, both physically and emotionally? Did the patient feel like it was a caring experience?

We also have to look at children leaving our school systems. Do our children understand basic concepts in physical and mental health? Do they know the basics of first aid or how to put feelings like anger or sadness into words?

In other words, a successful health system must center around the well-being of the consumer. That means focusing on the well-being of the people.

Measure What Matters

I have visited hospital systems and felt overwhelmingly positive about the patient experience. There is nothing new about waiting for a doctor who may be slightly or extremely late. However, having a nurse offer to get me coffee is not only new but also unusual.

That experience made me feel like I mattered. Would I recommend that doctor and that hospital system to someone? Absolutely. It is worth the longer drive to get exponentially better care. Face it, it is almost a privilege to have that choice, access, and time.

The care is better because everyone in the system is trained in something that is antithetical to the vast majority of modern medicine: customer service.

Patient experience data has to be taken seriously. Are you having a great experience despite not feeling well, or is your experience not so great? What do we do when the experience is subpar? Who is accountable? Who holds health insurers accountable for the experience I have in dealing with them? Unfortunately, the answer is murky. No one. No one is specifically held accountable for the customer experience in healthcare.

What is my recourse as an individual when the insurance company gives me a baseless answer of "no" without a sensible justification? What does it say about the state of healthcare when a request is denied one month and then the same request is approved one month later? What is the rhyme or reason?

The industry excels at financial accountability. What's missing is accountability for the experience itself. Where is the responsibility for how people are treated, for the fear, frustration or dignity lost along the way? That is emotional accountability. If we believe it matters, we must ask: what would the metric be?

The common metric that should bind these sectors, which I cannot emphasize enough, is the reason the health system exists in the first place. The patient experience and patient outcomes should be a focal point.

Insurance companies are also responsible for outcomes, not merely for cost. If a longtime customer is supposed to have a colonoscopy every five years, the patient should receive a notification after five years. At the very minimum, the patient's primary care doctor should be notified.

"According to our records, it has been seven years since your last colonoscopy. We wanted to reach out to make sure that you are healthy and to schedule a colonoscopy with the provider who last performed this. In addition, here is a list of other providers who are included in our health insurance plan within your zip code."

The benefits of preventive care can be viewed as both empathetic and revenue-driven.

When building a health system, the most important question to ask should be, "How does this system reflect the needs of those I ultimately serve?" The purpose of the insurance company, hospital system, doctor's office, and pharmacist is to serve the customer, not my beneficiary, and not the patient. We are always people, sometimes patients.

For example, my local pharmacy, Boyt Drugs, is privately operated and not part of a mega chain. It is not uncommon for me to call when I am out of my medication and have the pharmacist focus on my health situation.

The pharmacist asks me, "Do you need it for tomorrow morning or tonight?" If I respond, "I could really use it tonight," he would say, "I will have it in your mailbox this evening. Are you going to be home later?" I respond, "Yes, I will. Thank you very much." That is service. The pharmacist is using the pharmacy as a service operation for the customer.

Let us not forget that pharmacists are highly trained, patient-facing health professionals. They do not have stethoscopes around their necks, but pharmacists are Doctors of Pharmacology, and they often know their patients' medical histories better than the treating physician.

My pharmacist could say, "I am a doctor. I do not drop off medications. I am not a delivery service." But pharmacists seek and are trained to serve, which is central to why they choose the profession in the first place.

My late psychiatrist father-in-law was an analyst at heart. He was known to ask very probing and core questions: "What motivates you to do that? He looked at the essence or the catalyst of what made you "you." He instilled in my wife the importance of the individual's connection to the community, to family, and to themselves.

As someone who married into a family steeped in mental health, I came to appreciate the tools that help us focus on relationships. I have seen how much stronger people and organizations can be when they place those connections at the center.

In my own career, I have been fortunate enough to work within businesses that faced significant challenges. Some needed to be turned around, and others had to be built from the ground up. None of that was ever done alone. I had help, guidance, and colleagues who carried the mission forward with me. Collaborative culture and energy were key to our communal success.

What always mattered most was not the structure of the business but its purpose. What are we seeking to achieve? What principles will drive success? How

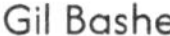

do we inspire people to want to work together for a larger cause?

This is the same question the health system must face. Payers, innovators, policymakers, and providers have not lost their calling because they lack compassion, but because the system often directs them toward priorities that seem almost contrary to their mission. At its core, the purpose is straightforward: to keep people healthy or restore their health.

The metrics, too, should be simple. Are fewer people sick? Are sick people getting healthier? How do people feel about their journey with us? Those questions have slipped from view as the system has begun to serve itself rather than the people it was created to serve.

Health systems that measure success by patient satisfaction outperform those that measure success by their bottom line. Doctors are far more enthusiastic about working in a system driven by patient satisfaction.

Mount Sinai in New York is led by Dr. Valentin Fuster, a physician whose presence lifts both colleagues and patients. A friend once shared how he spent more than two hours personally guiding her through complex care decisions. In another instance, he cleared his schedule to sit with a patient facing a difficult diagnosis, choosing to be fully present rather than handing the responsibility to someone else. These moments are not about prestige or position; they reflect his belief that every patient matters.

Imagine if that ethic became the blueprint for our entire health system. Not long ago, the doctor-patient relationship was deeply personal. Primary care physicians, cardiologists, pediatricians, and OB-GYNs often knew families well, sometimes even visiting them at home. Healing was not only about treatment; it was rooted in a relationship.

Systematization has given healthcare scale, but it has also weakened the personal bond between patient and doctor. Too often, people have become numbers. Population health is important, but it must never eclipse the person sitting in front of us.

Dr. Jeffrey Brenner showed how both truths can coexist. He approaches population health through households and individual needs, like the child with asthma who simply needs an air conditioner. He recognizes that while the system is vast, care must still be personal.

When medicine centers on people, the system comes alive. When it reduces people to data points, physicians risk becoming mechanics, fixing "brakes" as quickly as possible rather than restoring lives with care and purpose.

Today, the push is for throughput. Scraping data with AI helps the line move faster, but speed is not the same as healing. Anyone who has watched a production line knows the danger: the faster it runs, the easier it is for quality, safety, and human dignity to be lost.

To what end? To what purpose?

If you ask me about the purpose of medicine, the answer is simple: the purpose is to heal. We must connect healers with those who need healing. Health innovation is designed to support that purpose, not the other way around.

Gil Bashe

Integrate Advocacy into the Care System

Advocacy in healthcare has become particularly important for several key reasons. It provides a way for people to bond and to draw strength from others who are going through similar clinical journeys. These journeys may be connected by conditions such as asthma, cancer, allergies, psoriasis, or heart disease, for example.

Who did you see? What did you ask? In other words, advocacy was an early form of aggregating people's knowledge, creating a much-needed information support system. We are smarter together. Where gaps existed in addressing people's needs, groups were brought together. This led to fundraising drives for research and increased awareness.

Consider the impact women have had on reframing heart disease. Until the early 1990s, heart disease was still largely regarded as a man's condition, a misconception rooted in decades of research that underrepresented women, as Christine L. Miller, PhD, documented in her historical review, "The Evolution of Information on Women and Heart Disease 1957–2000" in Preventive Medicine.

The narrative began to shift in the mid-1990s, when the nationwide "A Difference in a Woman's Heart" campaign, supported by DuPont, the American Medical Women's Association, and the American College of Cardiology, initiated a long-overdue dialogue about women's cardiovascular risks.

I was privileged to contribute to that effort. Although credit is due to the many clinicians, advocates, and organizations that came together. Their efforts had a domino effect. That initiative sparked waves of conversation, drove new research, and began to change how the health community approached diagnosis and care for women.

It also showed the power of collaboration. When health innovation, professional societies, and patient advocacy align, the result is not simply heightened awareness but improved care. What began as a campaign became a catalyst, reminding us that advocacy is not separate from science; it is a partner in shaping it.

Patient advocacy remains essential, but it must evolve. The next phase is not only about demanding access to treatments; it is about insisting that the system prioritize the patient experience itself. People must speak with one voice to be treated not as cases or numbers, but as people.

Today, that voice is fragmented. Media report powerful stories of neglect or breakthrough, but one hospital's failure and another's success are seen as isolated. What happens at Hospital X or with Doctor Y is treated as anecdote, not evidence. Without a collective standard, no one is held accountable.

The answer is not more noise but a common voice, a voice that declares the system needs a common metric, and that metric is people's health and well-being.

Healing the system begins by restoring that focus. Patient experience, dignity, and outcomes must become the primary drivers of decision-making. When empathy

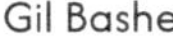

is the organizing principle, the money will follow, as trust and loyalty naturally follow.

At present, too much of the industry still asks, “How do we make sure we make money?” rather than, “How do we make sure we are focused on you?” It is time to reverse that equation. The patient must become the horse, and the system the cart, pulled forward by purpose, not weighed down by misaligned priorities.

Aligning Innovation with Impact

First and foremost, health innovation is a broad field. That is why I talk about multifaceted product innovation. Biological innovation occurs with gene splicing, gene editing, and CRISPR (Clustered Regularly Interspaced Short Palindromic Repeats), a clever acronym that describes a bacterial immune system designed to facilitate gene editing.

We are developing remarkable therapies for cancer and countless other diseases, and creating medicines and devices that address conditions long overlooked, such as neuropathy. Innovation is not our problem; it is happening every day. The real test is whether these breakthroughs reach the people who need them most, including those in economically challenged communities who are too often last in line for life-changing treatments.

At the same time, AI is transforming healthcare on multiple fronts, from guiding precision oncology decisions to reshaping clinical trial design, and from improving physician-patient engagement to streamlining operations. Yet concerns about AI misuse cast a long shadow over this promise. Large language models draw from vast pools of real-world data, but their "hallucinations" are not harmless glitches; misinformation can lead to dangerous outcomes, even contributing to crises like teen suicide.

The data feeding these systems comes from a wide range of sources: electronic health records, claims data, published research, patient-reported outcomes, payer policies, operational workflows, and digital interactions across the healthcare ecosystem. These are composite inputs—cleaned, coded, and analyzed, holding enormous potential for life-saving insights when used responsibly. It is time for health leaders to acknowledge that AI is already shaping hiring, training, and decision-making inside their organizations, and to confront both its power and its risks with equal seriousness.

AI is transforming public health by integrating social determinants of health, including economics and education, into predictive models. Companies such as Epic Health Research Network and Innovaccer are equipping health systems to anticipate and address community health challenges with greater precision than ever before.

"AI-driven insights empower health systems to deploy resources strategically, reducing disparities and improving outcomes across entire communities," wrote Dr. Michael Rosenblatt, scientist, teacher, former hospital president and medical school dean, former Chief Medical Officer at both Merck and Flagship Pioneering, and now Co-Chair of the Galien Foundation.

He also reminds us that sustaining breakthrough innovation requires aligning incentives with impact: "For companies to justify risking billions on finding a breakthrough drug, they need to be able to anticipate a corresponding return on their investment." His point is clear: profit and purpose are not adversaries; they are interdependent. Without financial sustainability, innovation withers. Without purpose, innovation loses its soul.

As some digital health pioneers, such as Daniel Kraft, MD, a digital health pioneer and founder of NextMed Health, shared in a 2025 interview with MobiHealthNews, "It's the ability to really bring healthcare anywhere. The ability to have basically an AI-enabled clinician and health coach on your smartphone... We can actually improve outcomes and lower costs and enable us to be much more proactive and preventative rather than reactive." His observations reinforce an essential truth: technology, when guided by empathy, amplifies human connection rather than eroding it. Yet it cannot replace human engagement, at least not yet.

The same principle applies to patient safety. Predictive analytics are transforming how risks are identified and addressed. Qventus, for instance, helps anticipate and mitigate perioperative complications. At the same time, companies such as Stasis Labs, Current Health, and Vytrac use real-time monitoring to send vital sign data directly to care teams. These insights enable earlier intervention and more confident clinical decisions.

As Amy Abernathy, MD, co-founder of Highlander Health and a former FDA official, shared in 2024, "Less than half of the (AI algorithms that we have available to us have been evaluated, and one of the challenges is they often have not been evaluated in our local clinical settings. So, we not only have to know that an algorithm performs as expected, but performs as expected here with my patients."

Her perspective underscores a larger theme: innovation is most powerful when it prevents harm before it occurs and strengthens trust between people and the system designed to care for them.

These advances remind us that health innovation is not abstract; it is saving lives and easing suffering. Consider psoriasis, a condition that impacts a person's sense of identity. For many, discovering effective treatment changes not only the course of the disease but also significantly improves their overall quality of life. Yet, awareness of these solutions differs by culture.

The Power of Asking Questions

In the United States, patients often learn about new therapies through direct-to-consumer advertising. This approach has an empowering effect, giving people the knowledge and confidence to ask treatment-related questions of their physicians. In Europe, the flow of information is reversed. The physician, acting as a trusted intermediary, typically introduces new options during the consultation. A doctor in Europe might say, "I see you're having a psoriasis flare-up. There's a new pill available. Take two of these each day, and in a month, we will see how it is working."

Both models aim to strengthen the connection between patient and physician, though in different ways. In the U.S., advertising encourages patients to be active participants in their care. In Europe, the emphasis rests on the physician guiding the conversation. Each reflects a cultural difference in how trust is built within the health system, and both underscore the importance of ensuring people feel informed, supported, and central to their own care.

I return here to patient advocacy because it is inseparable from the system's future. Advocacy organizations rally around people with shared concerns. They create spaces where patients can identify with others, share experiences, and feel heard. At their strongest, they expose the gaps in care and push for change, making visible what the system overlooks. That pressure is what drives new research, new treatments, and ultimately, a higher standard of care. Support groups do more than provide comfort; they have the power to transform the system itself.

We see this when payers create barriers. Advocates step in to help patients navigate a complex and often unyielding bureaucracy. In other cases, patients turn to one another in online forums and social media groups, trading insights on which doctors listen or which treatments have helped. What emerges is a powerful word-of-mouth network born out of necessity.

That necessity is central. People share their stories because the system does not make this knowledge accessible. So, patients create their own channels of wisdom. History shows that determined patient leaders can achieve remarkable results: they gather voices, curate knowledge, raise funds, and press for change.

This is both inspiring and sobering. It is inspiring because no one understands the patient journey better than those who are living it. It is sobering because the health system should not leave patients carrying this weight alone. The system exists for one reason: the patient. Advocacy fills the void, but the goal must be for the system itself to stand as a true partner in healing.

Communication as Part of Care

I believe that, fundamentally, communication should always be part of care. You might think that the implementation of care is the purpose of the system, or you might think that the purpose of the system is to maintain acceptable revenue streams. Either way, communication is part of care.

Awareness is a form of communication. By making people aware of how illness can arise within their bodies, we are communicating.

Education is a form of communication. Explaining to people why they have the illness or symptoms they have, outlining their options, and clarifying how their health insurance will or will not cover certain aspects of their care is effective communication. The connection between policy and health is communication. A doctor explaining preventative medicine to a patient is communication.

Communication is part of the "now." Physicians must maintain their zeal and passion for patient interaction.

Medicine is an interactive experience between the people seeking help, the people providing help, the people ensuring access to care, and the people we seek to invite into the system. Communication is part of care.

The problem is that physicians are increasingly drawn away from communication, which should always be part of care. Instead, they are thinking, "What do I need to do next?" The next person, the next treatment, and the next set of brakes that need to be fixed. Physicians are skipping over the "now."

Danny Sands, MD, and Mary Hennings of The Society for Participatory Medicine remind us that collaboration between clinicians and patients should not be an aspiration; rather, it is the foundation of better health outcomes. When care becomes a shared journey rather than a transactional directive, it closely aligns with patient expectations, enhances quality, and reduces costs.

However, collaboration remains more rhetoric than reality. The Society's late-2024 pilot survey, conducted in partnership with the Beryl Institute and Ipsos Pulse and involving 1,300 participants, offers a sobering snapshot of the current state of patient experience. More than half of the respondents reported that they did not always feel included in decisions about their care or that their clinicians were consistently honest with them. Only one in five felt regarded as experts in their own health, and trust was significantly lower among patients of color and those with limited incomes.

The findings expose a central pain point. The philosophical underpinnings of this approach were emphasized nearly 20 years ago in the Institute of Medicine's (IOM) report, Crossing the Quality Chasm. Patients who surrender the most control to clinicians often feel the least respected. This is not just a matter of bedside manner; it is a mirror held up to a system that too often values compliance over collaboration. Health is not something that is done to people. It is something built with them. Until clinicians and systems close the gap between care delivered and care experienced, the chasm between delivery and experience will remain a defining weakness of modern medicine.

Conversely, we are awash in information. Sometimes, it comes directly from the authorities. However, most often, the information comes through a media filter or an algorithm. It's all day, every day, and it's overwhelming.

To achieve strong communication, the messaging should be on point, ideally adhering to the three T's: transparency, truthfulness, and timeliness.

There is a fourth need that does not start with the letter "T." People need empathy and wisdom to guide them in their choice of words with patients.

A simple exchange of facts does not necessarily drive action. We do not emotionally trust facts. We either trust people or we do not. Moreover, we tend to trust authoritative voices proven to demonstrate powerful listening skills. As we process facts emotionally, we trust leaders who move beyond financial and medical data and speak to us in a voice that echoes how we feel in the current moment.

Everyone in the health system needs to remember their purpose. The receptionist sitting at the desk, the accountant paying the bills in a physician's office, the

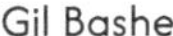

payer processing paperwork, the CEO of the world's biggest health insurer, the specialist, the primary care doctor, the nurse and the pharmacist, all of these people must say to themselves, "I have a purpose."

We must remember that sustaining life has a truly incredible and special purpose. As such, every action connected to care—our work, efforts, communication, touch, and decisions—carries weight. Even something as simple as saying, "I approve of this," or "I don't approve of this," has an impact. Remember, communication is always part of care. Is it meaningful? Is it helpful? Is it supportive? Is it caring? Does it lead to more communication?

Physicians or payers shouldn't make people feel like they have to say, "Okay, I get it," when they do not. Patients need to be invited to share what they don't understand or see as unreasonable. Otherwise, we ignore a wave of communication: "I don't feel heard. I don't feel cared for. I don't feel like I matter. I don't feel like I'm central. I feel peripheral." The current issue with the system is that communication is being minimized. The people we seek to care about sadly feel peripheral to the system.

This sense of alienation is at the core of the anger that boiled over in the case of Brian Thompson. When 26-year-old Luigi Mangione assassinated this health insurance executive, it was clear, whatever the justification, that he did not feel heard or cared for. He felt pushed to the periphery of the very system that was meant to serve him.

We see echoes of that frustration every day. A physician recommends a procedure, yet the insurer responds,

"We respect your doctor's judgment, but according to guidelines, this other treatment must come first." The patient explains, "That was already done last year under a different plan," only to be told to restart the process.

Perhaps the patient or doctor already knows that the prescribed treatment will not work due to a past reaction to a similar class of medication, for example. Savvy patients have told me that they will fill a prescription and not take a previous medication just so that they can demonstrate to the insurer that it has "failed." The cycle of appeals, denials, and shifting responsibility leaves people exhausted, angry, and convinced the system is indifferent to their suffering.

The comparison to retail is stark. If you return a sweater, you are not told to visit the shoe department and then the perfume counter before being helped. Yet in healthcare, people are routinely sent from desk to desk, office to office, insurer to provider, until their patience wears thin.

What makes this infuriating is not only the inefficiency but also the knowledge that the system is aware this is happening. Patients know they are caught in a loop designed to protect institutions, not to protect them. That awareness breeds despair and rage.

Communication must be treated as part of care itself. For medical professionals and system leaders, every denial, delay, or misdirection not only impacts health outcomes but also affects people's sense of dignity and worth. Patient care is not a transaction; it is a lifeline.

War is chaos. It is like an emergency room magnified many times over—smoke, shouting, blood, and the constant fear that another round of shelling could strike at any second. In that chaos, my mission was never in doubt: keep people alive. That was the purpose. Yet once a soldier, even an enemy soldier, was injured, they were no longer combatants. They became my responsibility—a moral obligation rooted in the code of conduct that defines who we are.

I vividly remember treating wounded enemy fighters. In those moments, I did not see ideology or a foreign uniform. I saw a broken body, terrified eyes searching for mercy. I felt their humanity touching mine, as if our lives were tethered together.

On the battlefield, there is no option to turn away. You have two choices: act to save a life or stand by and do nothing. No medic walks away to chase another firefight. You stay with the person in front of you because that is your duty, your mission, and your common humanity.

That choice separates true healing from mechanical maintenance. Lose that sense of awe, that recognition of humanity's divine spark, and health becomes nothing more than turning wrenches on a machine, another brake job on the line. Purpose keeps us from losing our moral clarity.

That same purpose must guide us beyond the battlefield. Whether you are in payer systems, administrative support, or maintenance, you are part of the same loop of care. A hospital that is not clean becomes a breeding ground for infections. We measure hygiene but rarely emotional hygiene, the atmosphere of respect, empathy, and dignity that also sustains health.

I grew up in a family that valued hard work, and my father set a great example. An auto mechanic, he was well-read, thoughtful, and precise, not unlike a surgeon who connects mind, movement, and mechanics. His craft was never just about fixing cars; it was about responsibility. He knew that when a family of five drove away, their safety rested on his work. Their lives were in his hands, and he carried that weight with quiet dignity.

The health system carries the same responsibility. I am calling for care that honors its purpose. Just as a mechanic must return a car with brakes people can trust, health professionals must deliver treatment people can trust.

Purpose and impact have two sides. We can do things on purpose, or we can act with purpose. We can cause an impact, or we can make an impact. That choice defines us.

My father never lost his sense of purpose, and that clarity gave meaning to every repair. Everyone in healthcare deserves the same clarity, to feel the weight and dignity of their role, to know that their work matters. When culture reminds us that healing is a calling, performance follows. That is how we revitalize the culture of health, inspire our people, and create innovations that truly serve.

Some in industry (though not all) have built the roof before laying the foundation, chasing priorities that leave people stranded in the desert with no oasis in sight. Yet, if we return to the purpose of holding lives in our hands, we can rebuild the system on solid ground and steer it back to what matters most: keeping people safe, healthy, and well.

Progress in the health sphere should not solely be about investing more money in innovation. We have to invest in people. More resources may mean more meaningful innovation, but at what cost?

Progress should be gained by focusing more on empathy. Who do we serve? Why do we serve? What is the outcome we seek?

Again, the pieces of our current health system often work at cross-purposes. Payers, providers, policymakers, and innovators circle one another in debate while life and death hang in the balance. Too often, it feels like this:

Provider, "I want to do this for the patient."

Payer, "I cannot authorize it without more justification."

Policymaker, "We must cut spending, even if it limits access for those in need."

Patient, "I'm rarely considered in decisions on which my life (or quality of life) depends"

In many ways, the physician is like Sisyphus, pushing the rock of advocacy up the hill repeatedly, only to watch it roll back under the weight of bureaucracy. In the end, who does that rock roll over? The patient.

This is not about villains and heroes. It is about empathy and communication, about remembering to ask, "How would I feel if I were in this position? How would I want to be treated?" The tragedy lies not only in denial or delay but also in the absence of a human connection in the decision-making process.

It does not have to be this way. If we can come together around a shared purpose, the outcome will be nothing short of life-altering.

Our collective voice must be clear: the purpose of the health system is to keep healthy people healthy and, to the best of our ability, return sick people to health.

When we unite around this simple, human truth, policies, practices, and innovations align. The system begins to serve its real purpose: people. That unity will bring lasting benefits to humanity, measured not just in years added to life but in dignity, trust, and wellness added to every life.

Ultimately, we all face mortality. What endures is not how long we live, but how we care for one another along the way, the health we restore, the compassion we extend, and the hope we inspire. This is the legacy we can choose to leave together.

THE NEXT CHAPTER BELONGS TO US

THE modern health system was not born of malpractice or neglect. It grew from good intentions, shaped by both its successes and its mistakes. Yet, like a city without a master plan, it sprawled unevenly, expanding where it could rather than where it should. There was no crystal ball. The system evolved without a clear, unifying blueprint.

All of us can look at the map of any major metropolitan city in America and question how it came to be. Why does this major thoroughfare into the city center have only two lanes? Why does this elevated train track run a few short feet away from someone's bedroom window? Why is there no green space in the heart of town?

The nation's vast medical infrastructure started as a small town that has grown into a bustling metropolis. The modern healthcare system is the product of historical evolution, economic pressures, social priorities,

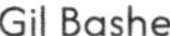

and contributions to biomedical innovation. The scope of what it would become could not be envisioned (nor predicted) when the first cobblestone was laid.

Like the reactionary evolution of urban development, medicine has needed to adapt to the times, react to unexpected detours, acclimate to budgetary realities, and accommodate all that could not be predicted, envisioned, or foreseen.

This fragmented approach has brought us to an era of gridlock in modern medicine. Little by little, it is pushing physicians to the periphery of health decision-making. Because the system is so massive and sprawling, it has forced entire sectors into silos as well. These silos compete for financial resources. This reality is at the center of any conversation on health kinetics.

It felt like forever before my daughter received an actual diagnosis. Nearly a decade ago, during her appointment with patient-centered cardiologist Nieca Goldberg, MD, something shifted. Dr. Goldberg did not dismiss my daughter's complex constellation of symptoms, nor did she refer her to yet another specialist who might not be reimbursable.

Instead, this physician said, "I don't know what this is, but we'll investigate."

"I don't know what this is, but we'll get to the bottom of it" is the most courageous response any medical professional can give today. This statement should be routine, but it is an oasis in our modern medical desert.

"I don't know what this is, but we'll get to the bottom of it," led to a workup that finally revealed the root causes of my daughter's illness.

"I don't know what this is, but we'll get to the bottom of it" centers attention not on the diagnosis or the symptoms, but on the patient's quest for answers.

"I don't know what this is, but we'll get to the bottom of it" is one of my metrics for determining whether patient-centered care is being offered.

There is too much focus today on profit and process for the system to consistently deliver patient-centered care. Whether it's the payer, the provider, the policymaker, or the product innovator, the focus is now on the process and payment. We must remember that, at all levels of the medical industry, patient care should be at the center of the conversation. In the beginning, the patient was the foundation of the practice of healing. This clarity has been lost.

There is an unspoken concern that if the patient's voice is prioritized, it will eclipse every other priority. That is not the case. Without profit, there is no sustainable industry. But without valuing the patient's experience, outcomes, and feedback, the industry loses its purpose. Both must exist, but purpose must lead.

The danger is clear. If we fail to elevate the patient's voice, we risk being forever gridlocked in the traffic jams of rapid change. We risk leaving silos intact, measuring budgets more carefully than lives, and forgetting the human being at the center of care.

Yet, the moment we decide the patient's voice matters, the system changes. The moment we decide the patient's data matters, the system changes. The moment we decide the patient's lived experience matters, everything changes.

I recently visited a new primary care physician. My longtime doctor had retired early, worn down by the endless demands of payer paperwork. My new doctor was kind, but our first visit lasted no more than 15 minutes; the allotted time before the next patient. My wife's first appointment with him lasted ten minutes.

In that short window, we covered the basics. However, no one asked about my fluctuating blood pressure or why my A1C sometimes rises and then falls back to normal. A simple question, "What happens when it goes up and what happens when it comes down?" could have opened the door to understanding my habits, my family history, and my risks. It might even have saved the system money and, more importantly, safeguarded my health. Instead, it was reduced to a checklist: review the file, check the medications, move on. Offering time is an expression of caring. I sometimes wonder what another ten minutes would truly cost or save.

That visit reminded me of the lessons my grandmother, who raised me in the deeper sense of the word, taught me. She was a survivor. Despite having lost her family at a young age, she carried no bitterness. She lived with persistence and love, never letting cruelty erase her humanity. From her, I learned that kindness is not weakness; it is strength. In war, in business, or in the ordinary struggles of daily life, kindness opens eyes and hearts. In healthcare, too, it is the spark that restores trust and connection. This is precisely what our system has lost and must reclaim.

Too often, we look for someone to blame, someone to "throw under the bus," to prove accountability. My grandmother taught me a different path: move forward, make things better, live for the future. That is what we need to do now.

Leaders across the health ecosystem, including payers, providers, policymakers, and innovators, all have the opportunity to embrace that same truth. Each can ask not only how to manage the system efficiently, but also how to make the future healthier. If we choose empathy and collaboration, we honor both the patient and future generations.

Where do we go from here? Rather than look for blame, we must now look to answer this key question. The goal is not to argue over whether payer, physician, or policymaker is right, but to focus on what will move us forward. Each side may feel certain in its position, yet resolution comes only when we return to the shared question that demands an answer.

We can't go down separate paths simultaneously. We recognize that the health system is both great and flawed at the same time. We recognize the enormous potential of artificial intelligence, large language model platforms, and other technologies to enhance the metrics of the health system. It is also terrifying.

Technology is not created in isolation from humanity. It amplifies our abilities. The biotechnology products we use were created by people, not machines. Medicines were created by people who had aspirations to help heal others. This is inherently embedded in the work.

Yet we often forget that these are inanimate tools. Whether it's a large language model or a pill designed

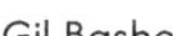

to treat a specific illness, each was created by people who aspired to heal. We tend to view them as passive objects, but they are, in fact, expressions of human intent. They are an extension of our drive to improve lives and, yes, to build sustainable businesses by doing good for others.

In my travels meeting innovators around the world, I'm reminded that most breakthroughs begin not in labs, but in lives. Entrepreneurs often introduce their companies with a personal story: a mother lost to breast cancer, a father nearly dying from an insulin overdose, a child facing a rare condition. Their work is born of love and urgency. I often tell them that investors may not care about those stories; money, after all, seeks money. However, we should care because those lived experiences are the true spark behind meaningful discovery. Innovation, at its core, is human.

Hyper-specialization is squeezing humanity out of the system. A doctor may treat one specific problem yet miss the broader context of a patient's life and health. This is a mistake. When we don't talk about (or respect) the humanity that went into creating medicine or technology, its greater purpose is lost.

My daughter's first gastroenterologist told her she needed another doctor; he was now limiting his practice to patients with upper esophageal issues. The next referral pushed her to a motility specialist. By the time she was shuttled to her fourth GI, that physician asked her why she had "so many gastroenterologists," as if the burden and the blame were hers. With each handoff, her humanity grew smaller in the system's eyes. Too often, we are no longer seen as whole people, but as collections of body parts to be divided, categorized, and dispatched.

Across the country, advocates like Rachel Lee step in where the system falls short, guiding people through a maze never designed with their realities in mind. Patients seek her out when no physician can see the full picture of their health challenges or when their lived experience is dismissed. Her gift goes beyond listening; she has the skill to recognize zebras when the system keeps insisting on horses. Yet the system rarely rewards the time and curiosity that kind of understanding requires. Patient advocates restore what too often goes missing: the partnership and presence that remind patients that their story still matters. Being seen and heard in today's care environment is becoming a challenge.

My previous primary care doctor spent some of her time looking at me and most of her time looking at her laptop screen, typing my responses to her required questions. Imagine if 90 percent of a doctor's attention were focused on you, the patient, the human being. This is where we have to envision our advances. The success of the medical industry must be about the people we seek to heal. It must be about harnessing technologies to improve efficiency, effectiveness, and human experience. These are not mutually exclusive.

In a period marked by intense partisan division, laws enacted in 2025 are expected to leave as many as ten million people without access to the Medicaid care benefits upon which they rely. Regardless of who is for or against a specific position, the reality remains: people

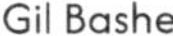

will still get sick. The urgent question is what happens when those who lose Medicaid coverage still need care.

When I consider that, I ask: Are we considering the impacts of our actions, inventions, ideas, or policies? Are we thinking about these decisions in terms of the actual effect on people's well-being and lives?

When we create injustice in the health system, we damage more than our capacity to help people get healthier. We send a message that the system has grown to sustain itself rather than us. It was not intentionally built to harm, but over time, its structures have favored efficiency, profit, and institutional survival at the expense of people. That message breeds disconnection, erodes trust, and undermines the belief that healthcare should exist to sustain and save lives.

We must create a new guiding principle. Are we making decisions that will save and sustain people's lives? Are we making people healthier in the long term, so they can be more productive and cost us less overall? Will our efforts advance that cause? Is this a refusal to adopt a shared principle, or is it another stumbling block placed before the blind?

Our medical schools train doctors using the same processes and procedures that were taught 20 years ago. Given the potential of AI technologies, how much do doctors truly need to memorize? How much fluency do doctors need with technological tools? Could we allow doctors to be more effective healers by freeing them to ask more questions?

All of these questions lead to a bigger question: Are we creating a society that maximizes humanity's and our inventions' greatness, or are we creating innovations that exceed our cognitive capacity to harness their full potential?

My friend John Nosta, a noted innovation theorist, suggests that as we make progress with large language models, we are ushering in "the death of I don't know." He asks, "Is AI making us smarter or just more certain?"

When I talk about empathy, I'm asking, "Is this the best we can do? Is this the best we can give? Is this the best we can receive? Is this the best we can pass along to future generations?" I am referring to a new frontier of mindfulness that enables us to reconnect with our shared humanity and humility, rather than being robotic.

There are many great doctors who have received countless accolades. Meet them in person, and you often find they are also remarkably humble, authentically centered on their mission. They may be accomplished and prosperous, but what stands out to patients and colleagues alike is their devotion to helping others live life to the fullest.

The best physicians are not motivated by titles or trappings. Their measure of success is far greater: "What will my impact be on the lives of the human beings I serve?"

Empathy is not about feeling good, doing good, or being good. It is centered in purpose, combining all of these. The empathetic physician places the patient at the core and asks, "What can I do better, or differently, to sustain life and restore health?" This question is key.

Technology, data, and protocols are only tools. Those tools help physicians meet patients' needs and inspire patients to take an active role in their own health. The

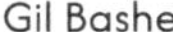

goal is not to check boxes; it is to create lasting outcomes: healthier lives, renewed trust, and human dignity.

Some of the greatest doctors I work with are well-known, well-respected heads of hospital systems, inventors, or department chairs. They don't see having 'Dr.' in front of their name as a tool intended to earn respect. They should be respected because they are offering help.

Sometimes, the greater the leader, the more humble the leader. The more they focus on culture, the more they focus on the impact their actions have on the lives of individuals. I have seen this truth embodied not only in my own family but also in leaders I deeply respect.

Peter Finn, Founder and CEO of FINN Partners, is a leader of distinction. In less than two decades, he has built one of the world's largest independent communication agencies. Yet his true achievement is not scale, but vision. From the start, he set out to create "an agency with a heart and conscience." His decisions center on values. He has demonstrated that empathy and collaboration are not merely soft skills but forces that unlock collective greatness.

I have been blessed with a life that has drawn together heart, gut, and soul alongside the practical realities of medicine and leadership. It has allowed me to view the health system from various vantage points. When I discuss being a combat medic, it may evoke an image of someone carrying a backpack of medical supplies in the field. However, my training and service also included hospital rotations. It is another perspective that shaped how I understand purpose, responsibility, and care.

I worked in the emergency room. I helped in gastroenterology and participated in surgical procedures. When I was brought in from the field, I observed everything. I observed how patients are treated, how they are received, how their needs are addressed, where equipment is stored and why, how instruments are used, why they are used, and what happened when they were used.

I also saw that different doctors had different mindsets. Surgeons felt like they had to cut to be validated. The specialists, who may have been in the ER as general physicians, were less interested and engaged if the procedure didn't involve their specific specialty. Based on my observations, they tend to be more interested in the body part than in the person.

Throughout my career, I have had several roles that offered a shift in perspective. As a lobbyist, I watched how policy decisions were made and how strategies were shaped by competing interests. In building health brands, I saw the raw emotions of patients and caregivers and came to understand that advocating with conviction was often essential to making treatments accessible and meaningful. In private equity, I witnessed how capital was deployed to build and sustain businesses and how access to funding often determined which innovations ever reached patients.

At every stage, I saw that facts were often secondary to opinions. Too often, power, perception, and convenience carried more weight than the well-being of people.

As the father of a child with a rare disorder, I know how hard families must fight to get the system to act. Through my wife's persistence in advocating for her parents and our daughter, I saw firsthand how patients

are often limited not by medical possibilities but by coverage caps, denials, and systemic shortcuts. The stress of waiting, the hours spent on the phone, and the constant push for approval weigh heavily on families already carrying the burden of illness. Advocacy becomes more than persistence; it becomes survival, the only way to turn possibility into care.

My father-in-law, a physician, often said, “I recognize the symptoms. But what is the root cause?” That wisdom applies not only to individuals, but to the health ecosystem itself. The root cause of the challenge is not fragmentation alone. Sectors drift apart or collide for a reason. They lack a shared goal. Let us start with people’s experiences and outcomes.

We must work together to improve the time human beings spend on this planet. We must train those leading our systems to have a better sense of self-awareness and empathy for the patient’s experience and needs. That voice, that need, that urgency is shared by each of us differently, but we all need to work individually and collectively toward the same mission—recognizing that people matter and the money follows that mission.

We are living through a time of tremendous cultural upheaval, driven by rapidly accelerating technology. Each advance, whether in the lab or at the coding bench, brings new costs and exposes the limits of outdated infrastructure. Many of our hospitals were built a century ago, yet they are expected to support 21st-century medicine. To deliver care that matches today’s innovation, we must also find the resources to renew the systems and spaces in which that care takes place.

The global population stands at more than 8 billion people. India and China alone each have more than 1.4 billion people. Health systems that were designed for far smaller populations between World War II and the 1990s now strain under the weight of unprecedented demand. Remote technologies are no longer optional; they are essential for scale and efficiency. Still, scale must not come at the cost of our humanity.

Medicine has always been about people. Medicine has held a sacred role since the 13th century. The earliest healers had no advanced tools. What they had was presence, compassion, and humanity. Today, we must ask urgently: Who still has time for bedside manner? Can that skill even be an option?

Technology should bring us closer to the healing tradition, not pull us away from it. Its greatest promise is to create space for clinicians to connect, listen, and truly care. That promise extends beyond the bedside. Innovators, too, must engage patients directly, listening to their needs and grounding invention in lived experience.

Real-world data essentially asks people to share a critical chapter of their lives. The accounts may be imperfect or even contradictory, yet together, they weave a vital thread of truth. Too often, the system dismisses these voices as outliers. We cannot afford to ignore them. Healing begins when every experience is valued, and when technology amplifies humanity rather than replaces it.

Regulators such as the FDA wrestle with this tension. They acknowledge the importance of patient-reported experience yet simultaneously downplay it at times.

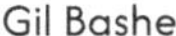

This inconsistency highlights a broader issue: How do we integrate the patient's voice into the system's design?

Consider long-term care facilities. They are often built for caregivers, designed to reassure children that their parents or grandparents will be safe. However, the residents themselves must also be heard. The facility should serve the people who live there, not just those who visit.

Too often, our decisions are made in isolation from the people we serve. As medicine becomes increasingly specialized, the whole person often disappears. My 93-year-old mother-in-law was recently told by an orthopedist, "It's good you're here for your hip area; I don't deal with knees and ankles." It's akin to my daughter needing to find a new GI because the current one now "only deals with the esophagus." You can't make this stuff up.

If this trend continues, many additional health factors may go unaddressed. Hyper-specialization squeezes humanity out of care. This is precisely where technology can help, if used wisely.

New AI diagnostic systems enable doctors to consider multiple symptoms simultaneously and identify possible conditions, including rare ones. This could help clinicians work more efficiently and with greater accuracy. We need to give physicians the time to use these tools well. Who will ensure they are trained to integrate technology into human care, rather than replace it?

At a recent conference, one attendee put it plainly: "You're right, but we'd need to add another year to medical school to train doctors on these tools." Perhaps it is time to revisit a decades-old curriculum. Just as important, we must prepare physicians emotionally for a high-tech world where their human connection may matter more than ever. Moreover, the urgency is real: patients are already uploading their own data, turning to generative AI for answers, and walking into clinics with a self-diagnosis in hand. Both doctors and patients must adapt quickly because the future of care is not waiting.

What's going to happen when a patient says, "Now that I have access to my EMR, I'm going to take the data and dump it into an OpenAI system and see what I have. Am I being treated correctly?" The system must examine what happens when we democratize information. What does that mean, and how do we deal with it?

Can I develop technology to help you become a better thinker, writer, or analyst? Not easily. I can provide you with tools to accelerate your process, but you still need to utilize your own cognitive talent. The same is true for medicine. Tools can be used to enhance effectiveness during the patient intake visit, but the patient still needs to connect with the physician. This is the human component.

Many years ago, a widely used blood glucose monitor was discovered very early on to have a calibration flaw. For patients relying on it, accuracy was a matter of daily health and safety. The company could have focused on legal or economic implications, but instead it chose a different path—one centered on the user experience. I was part of that process.

The company immediately recalled the faulty devices and replaced them with a proven, older model, along with free test strips, to ensure no disruption in care. Then, once the issue was entirely resolved, patients were provided with a state-of-the-art monitor with flawless calibration. At every step, the communication was clear, direct, and empathetic. Health professionals and patients alike praised the company for its responsiveness and integrity.

That moment stands out as proof that even in crisis, the right response is not to retreat behind lawyers or accountants. It is to meet people where they are with honesty, accountability, and respect. The lesson is simple: when you place patients at the center, trust follows.

The company could have chosen silence or legal deflection, but instead it chose humanity. The message was simple: “We’re sorry. We’ve identified the problem and taken immediate action to protect patients. Here is what we are doing to ensure you have accurate tools today, and how we will provide you with the most advanced solution tomorrow.” That clarity mattered as much as the technical fix.

What impressed me most was the willingness to lead with empathy. The company did not speak as a faceless corporation. It spoke as people who understood what it meant for patients and families to rely on their products every single day. That honesty transformed what could have been a crisis into a moment of trust-building.

Too often, our health system hides behind layers of lawyers, regulations, and protective language. Yet real progress comes when we remove the armor and connect as people. Empathy is not weakness; it is strength. It is the force that makes collaboration possible and keeps health systems worthy of people's trust.

If physicians are to give their best to patients, they need the backing of payers. If payers want people to believe the system exists to help them, they must engage in ways that affirm dignity and reduce frustration. When patients no longer have to battle the very system designed to serve them, adherence and outcomes improve. Overall costs decline.

In the middle of this maze sits another layer almost invisible to the public: pharmacy benefit managers, best known by the initials PBMs. PBMs negotiate formularies, rebates, and pricing structures so complex that even pharmacists struggle to explain them.

Patients often discover that a discount card from a service like GoodRx offers a lower price than their own insurance plan, an irony that highlights the system's opacity. Pharmacists tell me that they sometimes use these discount tools quietly, out of kindness, simply so patients can afford their medications. Yet corporate mergers and shrinking reimbursements have strained this relationship. Many pharmacies have stopped carrying certain medications because they incur a loss every time they dispense them. Another fracture appears: the trusted pharmacist, once a community anchor, is being pushed further from the patient by forces the patient never sees.

I have witnessed situations in which pharmaceutical and medical device companies are willing to sell their medicines for less, yet PBMs, whose compensation is often tied to the "savings" they negotiate, insist on a higher list price that can later be discounted. It is a dynamic that leaves patients confused (and scared), drug developers frustrated, and pharmacies caught in the middle. It is another example of a system that has grown so complex that the financial incentives often clash with the medical needs of the people it was designed to serve.

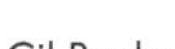

Pharmaceutical companies are also beginning to recognize that traditional drug distribution and reimbursement systems no longer reach everyone who needs care. As PBMs increasingly shape what patients pay at the pharmacy counter and which medicines are even available, drug makers are rethinking how their therapies reach people.

Increasingly, companies are exploring direct-to-patient pathways, an idea accelerated by the rise of Mark Cuban's Cost Plus Drug Company, which bypasses PBM go-betweens and insurers. This approach demonstrates that with transparent pricing, it's possible to simplify supply chains, reduce costs, improve access to essential medications, and treat patients as the central customer in the health ecosystem.

Policymakers, too, must recognize a simple truth: everyone grows old, everyone faces illness, and poverty magnifies vulnerability. We can choose to address these realities with foresight and compassion now, or we will pay a far greater price later.

Most health professionals enter the field of medicine with a desire to help people. We should place them in positions where they can fulfill that calling. Human connection restores value to their work and purpose to the system.

The danger is obvious: the more medicine resembles a conveyor belt, the less rewarding it becomes for professionals and patients. Without some change, more professionals will leave the system, or fewer will choose to enter. Some specialties already have shortages. The more patients avoid the system, the worse their health status. That is not the future we should accept.

Years ago, in another part of my career, I wrote about the power of emotion in shaping how people relate to brands. What distinguished the exceptional ones was not their feature set but their ability to make people feel seen and understood. Our health system stands at a similar inflection point now. We continue to add technology to a foundation that has never been properly repaired. The real transformation will begin only when we rebuild the human bond at the center of care. Connection, not complexity, is what ultimately heals.

How do we return to our original purpose of healing one another? Are we building a society that magnifies humanity's greatness in its approach to health? Can doctors once again have the time to sit with patients and listen? Who do we truly serve? What outcomes do we seek? Where do we go from here?

We put people on the moon. We have taken on moonshots in science, technology, and medicine that once seemed impossible. With all its brilliance and complexity, the health system holds the same potential. It does not need to be torn down; it needs fuel: empathy, collaboration, and a sense of purpose. With those, promise becomes progress. With those, we keep people healthy, return the sick to health, and measure success not only in years of life but also in the dignity, compassion, and hope we extend along the way.

That is the future before us. The answers are not yet fully written, but they are within our reach if we work together to find them. The next chapter belongs to us.

GIVING BACK: PURPOSE IN ACTION

THIS book was written with one purpose: to help heal the system that too often treats illness but forgets the person seeking care. Every story shared and every insight explored carries the same intention: to connect empathy with action.

In that spirit, 100 percent of my author royalties will be donated to not-for-profit organizations that embody the mission of this work. These include the Catskill Mountain Foundation, which demonstrates how the arts and community can revitalize both body and spirit; the Marfan Foundation, which supports patients and families navigating rare conditions with courage and grace; and Pinksocks, which reminds us that kindness, connection, and shared humanity are the true foundations of health.

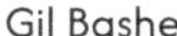

Your choice to purchase this book is more than an act of reading; it is an act of joining. You are part of a growing movement to reimagine how we care for one another. Each page you turn helps fund hope, creativity and compassion in action.

Together, we can prove that empathy is not a weakness in our system; it is its greatest strength.

About the Author

Gil Bashe is Chair of Global Health and Purpose at FINN Partners, one of the world's largest independent communications agencies. His path to health-sector leadership began on the battlefield, where he served as a combat medic in an elite paratrooper unit. The experience of tending to the wounded under fire shaped a career dedicated to connecting people with the care and innovation they need.

Over the course of four decades, Gil has served as an industry lobbyist, C-suite counselor, agency CEO, private equity executive, and advocate for patient-centered care. He has been listed among "The Top Brains in the New World of Work" by Fast Company, recognized by the PRSA Health Academy for "Excellence in Public Relations," and selected for the PR News "Hall of Fame." PRWeek named him one of the Top 30 Most Influential People in Health PR, PRovoke Media recognized him among their Innovator 25 communication leaders, and PM360 honored him with its Lifetime Achievement Award.

He serves on the boards of the American Diabetes Association and the Marfan Foundation, is an advisor to Let's Win for Pancreatic Cancer, and sits on several early-stage health company boards as a strategic advisor. Additionally, he serves as the editor-in-chief of Medika Life. As a Prix Galien Award Judge for The Galien Foundation, he helps recognize innovations that advance human and planetary health.

Through it all, his focus remains unchanged: ensuring that patients and their communities have a voice in their own care.

www.ingramcontent.com/pod-product-compliance
Lightning Source LLC
Chambersburg PA
CBHW042120190326
41519CB00031B/7556
9781613431818